In A Page
Neurology

Jon Brillman, MD, FRCPI
Chairman of Neurology
Allegheny General Hospital
Pittsburgh, Pennsylvania
Professor of Neurology
Drexel University College of Medicine
Philadelphia, Pennsylvania

Scott Kahan, MD
Series Editor

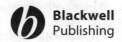

Blackwell
Publishing

© 2005 by Blackwell Publishing

Blackwell Publishing, Inc., 350 Main Street, Malden, Massachusetts 02148-5018, USA
Blackwell Publishing Ltd, 9600 Garsington Road, Oxford OX4 2DQ, UK
Blackwell Publishing Asia Pty Ltd, 550 Swanston Street, Carlton, Victoria 3053, Australia

05 06 07 08 5 4 3 2 1

ISBN-13: 978-1-4051-0432-6
ISBN-10: 1-4051-0432-5

Library of Congress Cataloging-in-Publication Data
In a page. Neurology / [edited by] Jon Brillman.
       p. ; cm.
   Includes index.
   ISBN-13: 978-1-4051-0432-6 (pbk.)
   ISBN-10: 1-4051-0432-5 (pbk.)

   1. Neurology—Handbooks, manuals, etc.
     [DNLM: 1. Nervous System Diseases—Handbooks. 2. Diagnostic Techniques,
Neurological—Handbooks. WL 39 P132 2005] I. Title: Neurology. II. Brillman, Jon.

     RC343.4.I5 2005
     616.8—dc22

                                                               2004027029

A catalogue record for this title is available from the British Library

Acquisitions: Beverly Copland
Development: Kate Heinle
Production: Debra Murphy
Cover design: Gary Ragaglia
Interior design: Visual Perspectives
Typesetter: TechBooks in New Delhi, India
Printed and bound by Sheridan Books in Ann Arbor, MI

For further information on Blackwell Publishing, visit our website:
www.blackwellmedstudent.com

Table of Contents

Table of Contents

Table of Contents

Table of Contents

Table of Contents

Abbreviations

AAA	abdominal aortic aneurysm	EEG	electroencephalogram
ABCs	airway, breathing, and circulation	EEG	electroencephalography
ACA	anterior cerebral artery	EMG	electromyogram
ACE	angiotensin-converting enzyme	ENT	ear, nose, and throat
ACTH	adrenocorticotrophic hormone	ESR	erythrocyte sedimentation rate
ADC	AIDS dementia complex	FSH	follicle-stimulating hormone
ADC	apparent diffusion coefficient	GBS	Guillain-Barré syndrome
ADEM	acute demyelinating encephalomyelitis	GCS	Glasgow coma scale
A-fib	atrial fibrillation	GERD	gastroesophageal reflux disease
ALS	amyotrophic lateral sclerosis	GI	gastrointestinal
ALT	alanine aminotransferase	HSV	herpes simplex virus
ANA	antinuclear antibody	HTLV	human T cell lymphocytotrophic virus
AQM	acute quadriplegic myopathy	HTN	hypertension
ARDS	acute respiratory distress syndrome	IBD	irritable bowel disease
AST	aspartate aminotransferase	ICP	intracranial pressure
AV	arteriovenous	ICU	intensive care unit
AVM	AV malformation	IM	intramuscular
BPH	benign prostatic hypertrophy	IV	intravenous
C-ANCA	cytoplasmic-antineutrophil cytoplasmic antibodies	IVIG	intravenous immunoglobulin
CABG	coronary artery bypass graft	LBP	low back pain
CADASIL	cerebral autosomal-dominant arteriopathy with subcortical infarcts and leukoencephalopathy	LDH	lactate dehydrogenase
		LES	Lambert-Eaton syndrome
		LFT	liver function test
		LH	luteinizing hormone
CCTV	closed circuit TV (monitoring)	MAO	monoamine oxidase
CBC	complete blood count	MCA	middle cerebral artery
CHF	congestive heart failure	MELAS	mitochondrial encephalopathy, lactic acidosis and stroke-like syndromes
CIDP	chronic immune demyelinating polyneuropathy		
CIP	critical illness polyneuropathy	MERRF	myoclonus epilepsy with ragged red fibers
CK	creatine kinase	MGUS	monoclonal gammopathy of undetermined significance
CJD	Creutzfeldt-Jakob disease		
CMT	Charcot-Marie-Tooth syndrome	MI	myocardial infarction
CMV	cytomegalovirus	MRA	magnetic resonance angiography
CN	cranial nerve	MRC	Medical Research Council (scale)
CNS	central nervous system	MRI	magnetic resonance imaging
COPD	chronic obstructive pulmonary disease	MRV	magnetic resonance venogram
		MS	multiple sclerosis
CPAP	continuous positive airway pressure	Na-K	sodium-potassium
		NF	neurofibromatosis
CSF	cerebrospinal fluid	NCS	nerve conduction study
CT	computerized tomography	NIHSS	National Institutes of Health Stroke Scale
CTA	computerized tomography angiography		
		NPH	normal pressure hydrocephalus
CVA	cerebrovascular accident	NSAID	nonsteroidal anti-inflammatory drug
DCCT	Diabetes Control and Complications Trial		
		OCP	oral contraceptive pill
DIC	disseminated intravascular coagulation	OPCA	olivopontocerebellar atrophy
		pCO_2	partial pressure of carbon dioxide
DM	diabetes mellitus	PCR	polymerase chain reaction
DVT	deep venous thrombosis	PML	progressive multifocal leukoencephalopathy
DWI	diffusion weighting image		
ECG	electrocardiogram	PMN	polymorphonuclear cell

Abbreviations

PNS	peripheral nervous system	SSPE	subacute sclerosing panencephalitis
PT/INR	prothrombin time international normalized ratio	SSRI	selective serotonin reuptake inhibitor
PTT	partial thromboplastin time	SVT	supraventricular tachycardia
PUD	peptic ulcer disease	TB	tuberculosis
RA	rheumatoid arthritis	TEE	transesophageal echocardiogram
RBC	red blood cell	TIA	transient ischemic attack
REM	rapid eye movement	TSH	thyrotropic-stimulating hormone
RPR	rapid plasma reagin	TTE	transthoracic echocardiogram
SAH	subarachnoid hemorrhage	tPA	tissue plasminogen activator
SBP	systolic blood pressure	U.S.	United States
SIADH	syndrome of inappropriate antidiuretic hormone	UTI	urinary tract infection
SLE	systemic lupus erythematosus	VP	ventriculoperitoneal
SNAP	sensory nerve action potential	VPL	ventroposterolateral
SOD	superoxide dismutase	V/Q	ventilation-perfusion ratio
SS-A	anti-Ro antibodies	WBC	white blood cell
SS-B	anti-La antibodies		

Assistant Editor

Lawrence R. Wechsler, MD
Director, Stroke Institute
Vice Chair, Department of Neurology
Professor of Neurology
University of Pittsburgh Medical School
Pittsburgh, Pennsylvania

Contributors

Susan M. Baser, MD
Associate Professor of Neurology
Drexel University College of Medicine
Senior Attending, Neurology
Medical Director, Spasticity and Movement Disorder Center
Allegheny General Hospital
Pittsburgh, Pennsylvania

Patricia B. Jozefczyk, MD, FAAN
Associate Professor of Neurology
Drexel University College of Medicine
Director, Botulinum Toxin Treatment Center
Allegheny General Hospital
Pittsburgh, Pennsylvania

Lara J. Kunschner, MD
Assistant Professor of Neurology
Drexel University College of Medicine
Attending Neurologist
Director, Neuro-Oncology Center
Allegheny General Hospital
Pittsburgh, Pennsylvania

Sandeep Rana, MD
Assistant Professor of Neurology
Drexel University College of Medicine
Attending Neurologist
Allegheny General Hospital
Pittsburgh, Pennsylvania

Thomas F. Scott, MD
Professor of Neurology
Drexel University College of Medicine
Attending Neurologist
Allegheny General Hospital
Pittsburgh, Pennsylvania

Contributors

George A. Small, MD
Assistant Professor of Neurology
Drexel University College of Medicine
Director, EMG Laboratory
Director, Clinical Neurophysiology Fellowship
Director, Neuromuscular Division
Allegheny General Hospital
Pittsburgh, Pennsylvania

James P. Valeriano, MD
Associate Professor of Neurology
Drexel University College of Medicine
Attending Neurologist
Vice Chairman, Department of Neurology
Allegheny General Hospital
Pittsburgh, Pennsylvania

David G. Wright, MD
Assistant Professor of Neurology
Drexel University College of Medicine Philadelphia, Pennsylvania
Attending Neurologist
Clinical Director of Comprehensive Stroke Program
Allegheny General Hospital
Pittsburgh, Pennsylvania

Reviewers

Merrit Fajt, MD
PGY-1 Resident, Internal Medicine
Pennsylvania State College of Medicine
Milton S. Hershey Medical Center
Hershey, Pennsylvania

Marian Sampson
Class of 2005
Meharry Medical College
Nashville, Tennessee

Sneha Shah
Class of 2005
Rush Medical College of Rush University
Chicago, Illinois

Jignesh N. Shah
Class of 2006
University of Louisville School of Medicine
Louisville, Kentucky

Niti Tank
Class of 2006
University of Medicine and Dentistry of New Jersey
Newark, New Jersey

Brenna Yard
Class of 2006
Wake Forest University School of Medicine
Winston-Salem, North Carolina

Preface

The *In A Page* series was designed to streamline the vast amount of material that saturates the study of medicine, providing students, residents, and health professionals with a high-yield, "big picture" overview of the most important clinical medical topics.

In A Page Neurology is the eighth handbook of this series. Neurology can be a complex and intimidating field of study. We have tried to cover the most clinically useful neurologic topics in a manner that facilitates easy understanding and quick retrieval of information. We expect this book to be especially useful for medical students, residents, physician assistants, nurse practitioners, and other health professionals.

As in the initial books of the series, we were often constrained by the size of the template and the need to keep each disease within a single page. We had to be quite succinct in our explanations and descriptions and we sacrificed details in some cases, such as drug dosages.

We are certain that the final product is a very effective resource. Reviews from medical students and residents have been very positive. We anticipate that this book will be a valuable tool in the hospital, as Board review, and for independent study. We welcome any comments, questions, or suggestions. Please address correspondence to drkahan@yahoo.com.

Acknowledgments

A heartfelt thanks to all contributors of this book and the staff of Allegheny General Hospital Department of Neurology. In particular, finishing this book would not have been possible without the help of Karen Less. We thank the staff of Blackwell Publishing, especially Kate Heinle. And we extend our love to Grace, Diane, Michael, Danny, Katie, and Julie Brillman.

The Neurologic Examination

JON BRILLMAN, MD, FRCPI

Section 1

1. Patient Evaluation & History Taking

History Taking

- A careful neurologic history is the most important factor in establishing the correct diagnosis and therapeutic course.
- History should be tailored to the portion of the nervous system involved.
- Unlike other medical specialties, anatomic localization is critical to establishing a diagnosis ("where" is often more important than "what").
- History should be evaluated in a chronological manner. Symptoms and complaints should be elicited by initial onset, time course, duration, progressive versus constant, and exacerbations/remissions.
- History must be obtained from family members or caregivers in patients with altered mental function or aphasia.
- Establish rapport with patient. Patients are often anxious and may have associated cognitive disorders.
- As in other specialties, the history largely dictates what diagnostic tests are necessary, if any.

Patient Evaluation

- The neurologic evaluation includes a thorough history, evaluation of mental status, and examinations of cranial nerves, motor system, sensory system, cerebellar function, reflexes, gait and station, and general medical examination as necessary.
  - History should include present illness with detailed evaluation of complaints and associated symptoms, past medical history and comorbid conditions (especially psychiatric disorders), past and present medications, family history (especially important in neurology due to the many inherited neuropsychiatric disorders), social history (determine habits such as alcohol use, illicit drugs, and smoking; relationships with spouse, significant others, and children; number of doctor visits; recent changes in life situations, and so forth), and be sure to determine and document handedness of patient.
  - In many cases, history should also be obtained from family members or caregivers.
  - Evaluation of mental status may include the Folstein mini mental status examination or a more thorough evaluation (see *Mental Status Examination*).
  - Evaluations of cranial and peripheral nerves, cerebellar function, reflexes, and gait should be evaluated (see individual entries).
  - Review old hospital records and reports from prior evaluations, examine prior X-rays and other imaging studies (reviewing images with patient and family members and explaining the significance of findings is very useful to establish rapport), and contact the patient's private physician or neurologist wherever necessary.
  - A focused general medical history and physical examination should accompany the neurologic evaluation as appropriate.
- Empathy and compassion are particularly important in neurology because of unfavorable prognoses in many conditions.
  - Living wills must be discussed in fatal conditions and code status in patients with conditions that may leave them in a vegetative state.
  - In cases of disorders with uncertain outcomes (e.g., multiple sclerosis), patients should be given favorable prognoses, wherever possible.
  - In terminal disorders (e.g., ALS, glioblastoma multiforme), assurance that the end of life will be made as comfortable as possible may calm patients' anxiety to some extent.
- Distinguish neurologic from psychiatric disease.
  - Neurologic and psychiatric disorders frequently coexist.
  - It is often difficult to distinguish neurologic from psychiatric disease. Requires an understanding of human nature, a knowledge of anatomy and physiology, and recogniton of emotional factors in individual patients.
  - Psychiatric causes of neurologic symptoms often represent attention seeking or conversion symptoms.
  - Depression often underlies neurologic disorders.
  - Anxiety exacerbates all neurologic signs.
  - Hysterical conversion symptoms and signs represent subconscious conversion of psychiatric features to physical signs.
  - Malingering represents a deliberate attempt of patients to fool the examiner or a conscious attempt to demonstrate deficit for secondary gain.
  - Signs and symptoms on exam that suggest psychiatric disease rather than neurologic disease include complete "give-way" rather than weakness on motor exam, weakness in a portion of extremity that does not conform to neuroanatomic patterns, complete analgesia instead of sensory diminution, complete loss of vibratory sense in an extremity, impairment of vibratory sensation on one side of jaw or nasal bone, and odd pitching and starting gait (pushing a leg or stepping and pulling a leg while walking).
  - Psychogenic coma may be uncovered by ice water calorics, which will move the eyes to the side of the ice water and nystagmus to midline.
  - Psychogenic seizures are writhing movements with pelvic thrusting and no post-ictal state.
  - Psychiatric disease is often a diagnosis of exclusion.
  - Imaging often necessary but may complicate management if unexpected findings or "red herrings" are present.
  - EEG may help differentiate seizures from nonepileptic seizures.
  - EMG and nerve conduction studies to determine if symptoms mimic peripheral neurologic disease.
  - Sedation or antidepressants, psychiatric consultation, and reassurance are often helpful.

2. Mental Status Examination

Level of Consciousness
• Assess level of consciousness: Alert and interactive, drowsy (falls asleep easily but responds to voice), stupor (does not respond to voice but awakes to painful stimuli), or comatose (no response to pain or voice).

Orientation to Person
• Assess orientation to person (identify self), place (identify location, city, country), time (year, month, day, date), and situation.

Memory
• Assess memory: Recent memory is tested by asking the patient to immediately repeat several digits or items. Recent memory can be tested by presenting several unrelated words or items and then several minutes later asking the patient to recite them. Observe if patient looks to spouse or other caregivers for answers.

Attention Span and Concentration
• Assess attention span and concentration by asking the patient to spell "WORLD" backward or count backward from 100 by 7s ("serial 7s"): 100, 93, 86, 79, 72 . . .

Behavior and Mood
• Assess behavior and mood by observing the patient's dress and appearance, alertness, irritability or agitation, attentiveness, interpersonal skills, and appropriateness of expressions to situation and questioning.
  –Abulia (apathy): Often reflects frontal lobe or pre-frontal lesions.
  –Aprosodia (flat affect): May indicate depression or frontal lobe lesion.
  –Inappropriate affect (e.g., excessive jocularity, inappropriate anger or hostility): May indicate frontal lobe lesion or early dementia.

Language
• Assess language by evaluating spontaneity and fluency of speech, reading and writing ability, comprehension of conversation, and ability to follow commands. Aphasia is the inability to convert thoughts into speech or inability to comprehend spoken language. It normally means damage to portions or all of the speech areas in the dominant hemisphere. Distinguish aphasia from dysarthria (impaired mechanics of speech, such as motor weakness of the tongue or lips). Loss of reading comprehension (inability to read and comprehend printed words) frequently accompanies aphasia and usually represents a lesion in the angular gyrus.
  –Nonfluent (Broca's) aphasia: Usually occurs with lesions of the frontal operculum (region where frontal and temporal lobe join). The patient uses few words, is easily frustrated, and uses frequent paraphasic errors (e.g., referring to a watch as a "time"). Often associated with mild contralateral hemiparesis. While the patient's speech is nonfluent, their comprehension is intact.
  –Fluent (Wernicke's) aphasia: Occurs with lesions in the superior temporal gyrus. The patient is verbose (words sound normal), but he makes little sense and answers not related to the questions asked. There is impaired comprehension. No associated weakness.
  –Conduction aphasia: Occurs with lesions of the arcuate fasciculus, a white matter band that connects Broca's area to Wernicke's area. Comprehension and repetition are impaired.
  –Global aphasia: The most common deficit. Represents lesions that involve both Broca's and Wernicke's areas. Patients are unable to comprehend language or speak fluently. Patients are often mute.
  –Transcortical aphasia: Generally occurs with subcortical lesions, resulting in defects of fluency or comprehension despite a retained ability to repeat words (e.g., ask patient to repeat "no ifs, ands, or buts").
  –Anomic aphasia: Impaired ability to name simple objects. Commonly seen in patients with dementia.
  –Alexia without agraphia is seen in nondominant occipital lesions and portions of corpus callosum.

Agnosia
• Assess for agnosia, the inability to recognize previously learned information.
  –Astereognosia (object agnosia): Inability to recognize objects by touch; due to inferotemporal lesions.
  –Prosopagnosia: Inability to recognize faces; due to bilateral parieto-occipital lesions.
  –Neglect: Ignoring a limb or half of the environment; due to contralateral posterior parietal lesions.
  –Anton's syndrome: Cortical blindness with denial of blindness; due to bilateral parieto-occipital lesions.
  –Balint's syndrome: Neglect of any object not fixated upon; due to bilateral parieto-occipital lesions.

Apraxia
• Assess for apraxia, the inability to perform or imitate specific movements despite intact understanding and being physically able to do so (i.e., intact strength and sensation). Usually reflects dysfunction of the parietal lobe. If the dominant parietal lobe is involved, apraxia may be masked by aphasia.
  –Ideational apraxia: Inability to stir a cup or use a toothbrush on command.
  –Dressing apraxia: Inability to put clothes on properly.
  –Constructional apraxia: Inability to copy simple designs.
  –Gait apraxia: Uncertain, clumsy steps; common in frontal lobe lesions.

3. Cranial Nerve Examination

Cranial Nerve I (Olfactory Nerve)
- ACTION: Governs the sense of smell.
- TESTING: Rarely tested in clinical practice; may be tested by asking the patient to identify several aromas; test each nostril separately; note that there is no cortical representation of smell, thus anosmia can be caused only by compression of the olfactory nerve, not by cerebral lesions.
- LESIONS: Meningioma of the olfactory groove, trauma.

Cranial Nerve II (Optic Nerve)
- ACTION: Vision and visual fields.
- TESTING: Evaluate visual acuity with Snellen chart and examine visual fields by finger movement.
- LESIONS: Ischemic, demyelinating, or compressive lesions of the optic tract or optic radiations.

Cranial Nerve III (Oculomotor Nerve)
- ACTION: Pupillary component (constrict pupil to light and convergence) and oculomotor component (innervates the levator muscle of the eyelid, superior rectus, inferior rectus, medial rectus, and inferior oblique muscles).
- TESTING: For pupillary component, check size, symmetry, and response to light, both directly and consensually, and check response to convergence. For oculomotor component, evaluate eye motion in all directions.
- LESIONS: Aneurysms or diabetic neuropathy are the most common lesions. If pupillary component is lesioned, the pupil will be dilated. If oculomotor component is lesioned, the eye will be deviated inferolaterally with ptosis of the eyelid.

Cranial Nerve IV (Trochlear Nerve)
- ACTION: Innervates superior oblique muscle, which depresses the eye when in the medial position of the orbit (downgaze with eye adducted).
- TESTING: Tested with cranial nerve III by assessing eye movement; evaluate for downward rotation of conjunctival vessels.
- LESIONS: Usually posttraumatic. When lesioned, patients will have vertical diplopia when looking down.

Cranial Nerve V (Trigeminal Nerve)
- ACTION: Motor component innervates muscles of mastication. Sensory component innervates the face.
- TESTING: Test by palpation with pin and light touch over face. Also test corneal reflex (touch cornea lightly with wisp of clean cotton, eyes will blink if normal).
- LESIONS: Brainstem glioma, brainstem infarct, multiple sclerosis.

Cranial Nerve VI (Abducens Nerve)
- ACTION: Innervates lateral rectus muscle.
- TESTING: Tested in conjunction with cranial nerves III and IV by observing motion of eyes in all directions.
- LESIONS: Diabetic neuropathy, increased intracranial pressure. Dysfunction results in medial deviation of the eye and diplopia.

Cranial Nerve VII (Facial Nerve)
- ACTION: Innervates muscle of facial expression.
- TESTING: Evaluate ability to close eyes tightly, smile, and grimace.
- LESIONS: Multiple sclerosis, Bell's palsy, stroke. Facial nerve dysfunction results in paresis of the face with inability to close eye.

Cranial Nerve VIII (Auditory and Vestibular Nerves)
- ACTION: Balance and hearing.
- TESTING: Test hearing by whispering to the patient; Weber test (place tuning fork on top of head) may localize lesion to the ear with conductive hearing defect; Rinne test (place tuning fork on mastoid process) also tests for conductive hearing defect.
- LESIONS: Acoustic neuroma. Dysfunction results in hearing loss, tinnitus, and imbalance with vertigo.

Cranial Nerve IX (Glossopharyngeal Nerve)
- ACTION: Taste sensation in posterior one-third of tongue; afferent component of gag reflex.
- TESTING: Test by inducing gag reflex. Touch palate with tongue blade and look for ipsilateral contraction.
- LESIONS: Lateral medullary stroke.

3. Cranial Nerve Examination

Cranial Nerve X (Vagus Nerve)
- ACTION: Swallowing, parasympathetic function to heart, efferent component of gag reflex.
- TESTING: Usually tested by inducing gag reflex. Touch palate with tongue blade, look for ipsilateral contraction.
- LESIONS: Lateral medullary stroke, recurrent laryngeal nerve lesions.

Cranial Nerve XI (Spinal Accessory Nerve)
- ACTION: Innervates sternomastoid muscle.
- TESTING: Tested by head turning and shoulder shrug.
- LESIONS: Tumors in the region of the foramen magnum.

Cranial Nerve XII (Hypoglossal Nerve)
- ACTION: Tongue protrusion.
- TESTING: Tested by observing tongue movements.
- LESIONS: Skull base metastases, meningeal carcinomatosis. Dysfunction results in tongue deviation to side of lesion.

- Lower cranial nerves receive bilateral innervation and are therefore only mildly involved with upper motor neuron lesions.
- **Pseudobulbar palsy** may mimic cranial nerve lesions: Denotes dysfunction of the brainstem resulting from bilateral upper motor neuron lesions (e.g., bilateral strokes), causing spasticity of swallowing and tongue movements with brisk jaw and gag reflexes and frequently emotional incontinence (e.g., inappropriate laughing or crying).

4. Motor Examination

Lesions of Upper Motor Neuron or Central Nervous System Result In:

- Weakness: In the upper extremities, weakness is characterized by drift of an outstretched arm on the contralateral side of the lesion, with extensors generally weaker than flexors. In the lower extremities, flexors are generally weaker than extensors.
- Muscle tone is increased to passive movement (spasticity); may exhibit "clasp-knife" effect; early pyramidal tract lesions may cause flaccidity, which then evolves to spasticity in a matter of days.
- Rigidity is an alteration in tone similar to spasticity, except that it is not dependent on rate of limb movement; commonly altered in extrapyramidal disorders (e.g., Parkinson's disease); not associated with increased reflexes or Babinski signs.
- Deep tendon reflexes are exaggerated (hyperreflexia).
- Pathologic reflexes are frequently present, including Hoffman reflex (increased finger flexor reflex) and Babinski signs.

Lesions of Lower Motor Neuron or Peripheral Nervous System Result In:

- Weakness is confined to the innervated muscles involved (e.g., ulnar nerve injury will involve most intrinsic hand muscles and flexor carpi ulnaris, peroneal nerve injury will result in foot drop).
- Muscle tone is always reduced (flaccidity).
- Fasciculations may be present.
- Deep tendon reflexes are always reduced or absent.
- Pathologic reflexes (e.g., Babinski sign) are not present.

Muscle Strength Scale (0–5)

0: Absence of muscle contraction
1: Muscle contraction is present but extremity cannot be moved
2: Some movement occurs but the patient cannot hold the extremity up against gravity
3: Extremity can be moved against gravity but not against external resistance
4: Able to move against some resistance
5: Full strength

Useful Myotomes

C5: Deltoid (arm abduction), biceps (elbow flexion)
C6: Wrist extension
C7: Wrist flexion
C8: Finger flexion
T1: Finger adduction and abduction
L1, L2, L3: Iliopsoas (hip flexion)
L2, L3, L4: Quadriceps (knee extension)
L5: Dorsiflexion, eversion, and inversion of the foot
S1: Plantarflexion
S2, S3, S4: External anal sphincter

Deep Tendon Reflex Testing

- Deep tendon reflexes tested generally include the supinator reflex (primarily C6—radial nerve), biceps reflex (primarily C5—musculocutaneous nerve), triceps reflex (C7—radial nerve), knee or patellar reflex (primarily L4—femoral nerve), and ankle reflex (S1—posterior tibial nerve).
  - Generalized hyporeflexia suggests peripheral neuropathy.
  - Unilateral hyporeflexia suggests radiculopathy, plexopathy, or mononeuropathy.
  - Hyperreflexia suggests upper motor neuron disease and generally associated with spasticity and Babinski sign.
  - Hyporeflexia of the upper extremities with hyperreflexia of the lower extremities suggests ALS or cervical spinal disease.
  - Babinski sign represents upper motor neuron disease but is normal in infants.
  - Jaw jerk should be tested if pseudobulbar palsy suspected.
  - Superficial reflexes (e.g., abdominal reflexes) may be absent in normal patients.

Reflex Scale

0: Absent reflex
1: Decreased reflex
2: Normal reflex
3: Increased reflex
4: Transient clonus (repetitive contractions of a hyperextended limb)
5: Sustained clonus

5. Sensory Examination

Assess Pain, Temperature, and Light Sensation
- Pain, temperature, and light touch are transmitted via the sensory nerve endings, spinothalamic tracts, ventroposterio-lateral (VPL) nucleus of the thalamus, and the post-central sensory cortex in the parietal lobe.
- Pain sensation is tested by use of a disposable pin. For CNS lesions, test entire side of body. With cortical sensory dysfunction, arm will drift aimlessly if outstretched. In cases of suspected spinal cord lesions, look for a sensory level (an area on trunk where there is a clear difference in sensation). For peripheral nervous system lesions, pin should be used over dermatome or distribution of peripheral nerve. Findings for temperature appreciation will be the same as for pain sensation.
- Light touch is tested by use of a finger or wisp of cotton. Rarely absent completely because of wide overlap in the sensory system.

Assess Vibratory and Position Sensation
- Vibration and position sense are transmitted via the sensory nerve endings, posterior columns of the spinal cord, medial lemniscus, thalamus, and sensory cortex.
- Vibratory sensation is tested by moving a tuning fork (128 Hz) over each joint, beginning with the toes.
- Joint position sensation is tested by moving a toe or finger rapidly and ask patient which direction the digit is moved. This is the ideal test for posterior column function.
- Romberg sign evaluates if the patient can remain steady while standing with eyes closed. Unsteadiness with eyes closed indicates dysfunction of large fiber peripheral nerves or the posterior columns in the lower extremities. Unsteadiness with eyes open suggests a cerebellar lesion.

Assess Cortical Sensation (Evaluates Parietal Function)
- Two-point discrimination test.
- Graphesthesia: Ability to identify numbers "written" on each palm with the examiner's finger.
- Topognosia: Ability to localize sensation (patient must determine where he is being palpated with his eyes closed).
- Stereognosis: Ability to identify shapes and sizes by touch (place objects in patient's palms).

Useful Dermatomes
C5: Shoulder
C6: Thumb and index finger
C7: Middle finger
C8: Ring finger and pinky finger
T4: Nipple line
T10: Umbilicus
L1: Inguinal region
L4: Top of thigh
L5: Dorsum of foot
S1: Plantar surface of foot
S2, S3, S4: Perianal

6. Cerebellar Examination

- The primary functions of the cerebellum are to maintain balance, posture, and coordination.
  - The cerebellar hemispheres dictate appendicular balance and coordination.
  - The cerebellar vermis dictates truncal balance and posture.
- The cerebellum may be damaged by atrophy (inherited, chronic alcohol use, paraneoplastic), multiple sclerosis, hemorrhage, stroke, or tumors (hemangioblastoma, medulloblastoma, astrocytoma, metastases).

Cerebellar Dysfunction

- Dysfunction of the cerebellar hemispheres results in incoordination of movement and speech.
  - Ataxia: Incoordination of trunk or limbs.
  - Appendicular ataxia: Patient is unable to perform finger-to-nose or heel-to-shin maneuvers.
  - Dysmetria: Inability to judge distances.
  - Dysarthria: Clumsiness of speech.
  - Past-pointing and rebound (overshoot and inability to check movements).
  - Dysdiadochokinesis: Defects in rapid alternating movements (rapidly tapping index finger to thumb, rapid pronation and supination of the forearm).
  - Imbalance of stance.
- Dysfunction of the cerebellar vermis (midline cerebellar dysfunction) results in truncal ataxia and may be observed during upright sitting or during ambulation.
  - Truncal ataxia: Staggering and pitching gait and titubation of trunk while attempting to walk.
  - Titubation: Oscillation of trunk and limbs.

7. Gait Examination

• Included in the examination of gait are posture, station, ability to stand from a seated position, and ambulation.

Posture

• Posture is analyzed for telltale discrepancies.
  – Patients with unstable posture may have cerebellar, basal ganglia, or labyrinthine disease.
  – Excessively erect posture is associated with progressive supranuclear palsy.
  – "Stooped" (universal flexion) posture is associated with Parkinson's disease.
  – Exaggerated lumbar lordosis is associated with proximal lower extremity weakness (e.g., muscular dystrophy).
  – Wide-based posture is often associated with cerebellar dysfunction.

Station

• Station refers to position of body during erect stance. Test with eyes open and closed.
  – Swaying with eyes opened indicates disorder of vestibular or cerebellovestibular system.
  – Swaying with eyes closed (Romberg sign) indicates dysfunction of large fiber peripheral nerves in the lower extremities or posterior columns.
  – Patients unable to stand on one foot may have cerebellar, basal ganglia, or labyrinthine disease.

Gait

• "Freezing" during gait or turning suggests basal ganglia disease.
• Slow ambulation or decreased stride length may indicate pyramidal or extrapyramidal disease.
• Patients with Parkinson's disease often exhibit a festinating gait of rapid, short steps and difficulty coming to a stop.
• "Steppage" gait (inadequate dorsiflexion resulting in exaggerated lifting of the affected leg during each step) may occur in L5 radiculopathy or common peroneal neuropathy.
• "Waddling" gait is seen with hip girdle weakness.
• Difficulty to walk on toes suggests S1-S2 radiculopathy or posterior tibial neuropathy.
• Gait apraxia (inability to walk normally despite intact strength) is seen in elderly patients with or without dementia. Characterized by small, uncertain steps with a tendency to fall. In late gait apraxia, patient may not be able to stand and feet may seem "magnetized" to the floor.
• Hemiparetic gait: Affected leg is circumducted with plantar flexion and inversion. Associated with any cause of hemiparesis or hemispasticity.
• Dystonic gait: Leg held in fixed posture and frequently dragged. Associated with torsion dystonia.
• Scissors gait: Thighs may rub together as there is powerful adductor spasm. Seen in bilateral hemisphere disease or spinal cord lesions.
• Parkinsonian gait: Small, shuffling steps with flexion of trunk and extremities. Tendency for propulsion and retropulsion.
• Ataxic gait: Broad-based gait with swaying, frequently with titubation. Associated with cerebellar disease.
• Posterior column dysfunction gait: Tends to be broad-based with legs lifted high when stepping.
• Steppage gait: Leg is lifted high to clear toe off ground in foot drop.
• Waddling gait: Pelvis and hips shift from side to side due to hip girdle weakness in myopathies (e.g., polymyositis).
• Hysterical gait: Pushing or pulling leg or staggering in various directions and pitching randomly.
• Choreic gait: Dancing type movements, frequently with toe walking. Seen in Huntington's disease.

8. Neurologic Localization

Central Nervous System (CNS)

• The CNS (upper motor neurons) includes the brain and spinal cord. Upper motor neuron lesions result in cognitive disorders, spasticity, hyperreflexia, sensory alterations, and pathologic reflexes.
  –Cerebral hemispheres
  –White matter tracts
  –Cerebellum
  –Basal ganglia
  –Brainstem
  –Cranial nerves I and II
  –Spinal cord
  –In general, cerebral lesions involving gray matter (cortex) are associated with defects in higher cortical function (e.g., dementia, aphasia) and seizures, whereas those involving white matter (subcortex) are associated with hemiparesis and hemisensory defects. Note that many lesions are mixed.

Peripheral Nervous System (PNS)

• The PNS includes lower motor neurons and the nervous system outside the CNS. Lower motor neuron lesions result in weakness, flaccidity, sensory alterations, and loss of deep tendon reflexes but absence of pathologic reflexes.
  –Cranial nerves III-XII
  –Spinal nerves and nerve roots
  –Cauda equina
  –Lower motor neurons, including anterior horn cells, nerve roots, peripheral nerves, neuromuscular junctions, and skeletal muscles
  –Plexuses

Frontal Lobe

• FUNCTIONS: Cognition, personality, speech, reasoning ability.
• COMMON LESIONS: Strokes, tumors, and trauma.
• LESIONS RESULT IN: Cognitive disorders (e.g., dementia), gaze deviation to side of lesion, abulia (slowness of response), nonfluent aphasia, hemiparesis, partial seizures.

Temporal Lobe

• FUNCTIONS: Memory and emotions.
• COMMON LESIONS: Tumors and trauma.
• LESIONS RESULT IN: Memory impairment, homonymous hemianopsia, aphasia (if dominant hemisphere), complex partial seizures.

Parietal Lobe

• FUNCTIONS: Sensation, praxis (ability to carry out desired acts).
• COMMON LESIONS: Strokes, tumors, and trauma.
• LESIONS RESULT IN: Hemiparesis, hemisensory deficits, apraxia (difficulty performing previously learned tasks), partial seizures.

Occipital Lobe

• FUNCTIONS: Vision.
• COMMON LESIONS: Strokes, tumors, and trauma.
• LESIONS RESULT IN: Homonymous hemianopsia or blindness.

Thalamus

• FUNCTIONS: Integration of sensory functions.
• COMMON LESIONS: Strokes, hemorrhage.
• LESIONS RESULT IN: Altered sensation and pain on opposite side, gaze deviation usually to side of lesion.

Internal Capsule

• FUNCTIONS: Pathway for motor and sensory systems.
• COMMON LESIONS: Strokes, hemorrhage.
• LESIONS RESULT IN: Contralateral hemiparesis and hemisensory deficits.

Cerebellum

• FUNCTIONS: Balance and coordination.
• COMMON LESIONS: Strokes, hemorrhage, and tumors.
• LESIONS RESULT IN: Ataxia, dysmetria, incoordination.

8. Neurologic Localization

Midbrain
- FUNCTIONS: Integration of vertical eye movements, sensory and motor functions.
- COMMON LESIONS: Strokes.
- LESIONS RESULT IN: Pupillary dilatation, paralysis, oculomotor weakness frequently accompanied by contralateral hemiparesis, tremor, or ataxia; paresis of upgaze.

Pons
- FUNCTIONS: Vital functions (e.g., breathing, consciousness, cardiac function), motor and sensory functions, lateral eye movement.
- COMMON LESIONS: Stroke, multiple sclerosis.
- LESIONS RESULT IN: Hemi- or quadriplegia, pinpoint pupils, horizontal gaze palsy, internuclear ophthalmoplegia, coma or "locked-in" state; upbeat nystagmus is common.

Medulla
- FUNCTIONS: Swallowing, cardiac function, balance, lingual movements, motor and sensory function.
- COMMON LESIONS: Strokes, syrinx.
- LESIONS RESULT IN: Lateral medullary or Wallenberg's syndrome (crossed sensory syndrome—numbness on one side of the face and the opposite side of the body), hoarseness, dysphagia, Horner's syndrome, and ipsilateral ataxia); medial medullary syndrome (ipsilateral tongue deviation and contralateral hemiparesis).

Cervical Spinal Cord
- FUNCTIONS: Sensory and motor function of arms and legs.
- COMMON LESIONS: Usually spondylosis (cervical degenerative joint disease), multiple sclerosis, trauma.
- LESIONS RESULT IN: Quadra- or paraparesis, spasticity in arms and legs with Babinski signs, sensory level in cervical area, urinary retention, loss of position sense.

Thoracic Spinal Cord
- FUNCTIONS: Motor and sensory function in legs, bladder function.
- COMMON LESIONS: Usually tumors metastatic to bone or intradural tumors (e.g., meningioma, neurofibromas); strokes and herniated disks are rare.
- LESIONS RESULT IN: Spastic paraparesis or paraplegia with bilateral Babinski signs; sensory level in thoracic area; urinary retention; loss of position sense in feet (unless anterior spinal artery syndrome, in which case posterior column function spared).

Conus Medullaris
- FUNCTIONS: Bladder and bowel function.
- COMMON LESIONS: Usually tumors in region of L1.
- LESIONS RESULT IN: Saddle anesthesia, bladder and bowel dysfunction, pain in legs may occur late in course.

Cauda Equina
- FUNCTIONS: Sensory and motor function in legs, bladder and bowel function.
- COMMON LESIONS: Usually herniated lumbar disks or meningeal cancer.
- LESIONS RESULT IN: Scattered pain and weakness in legs, loss of knee and/or ankle reflexes, bladder and bowel dysfunction.

Anterior Horn Cells
- FUNCTIONS: Motor function to individual muscles.
- COMMON LESIONS: Usually motor neuron disease (e.g., ALS).
- LESIONS RESULT IN: Weakness, flaccidity, fasciculations, and atrophy in the distribution of the motor unit, loss of reflexes.

Nerve Root
- FUNCTIONS: Sensory and motor function to individual muscles.
- COMMON LESIONS: Disk herniation.
- LESIONS RESULT IN: Usually causes pain and paresthesias in the dermatomal distribution and weakness in the myotomal distribution.

8. Neurologic Localization

Peripheral Nerve
- FUNCTIONS: Sensory and motor function to individual muscles.
- COMMON LESIONS: Usually peripheral neuropathies, solitary nerve or plexus lesions, or mononeuritis multiplex.
- LESIONS RESULT IN: Numbness, paresthesias, weakness, flaccidity, loss of reflexes, and loss of vibratory and position sense in the nerve distribution.

Neuromuscular Junction
- FUNCTIONS: Motor function to individual muscles.
- COMMON LESIONS: Usually myasthenia gravis.
- LESIONS RESULT IN: Variable weakness with fatigability; absence of sensory findings and normal reflexes.

Muscle Disease
- FUNCTIONS: Movement of joints and strength.
- COMMON LESIONS: Usually muscular dystrophies or polymyositis.
- LESIONS RESULT IN: Proximal muscle weakness with intact reflexes and absence of sensory symptoms or findings.

9. Neuroimaging

- Common neuroimaging modalities include X-rays, CT scanning, and MRI.

X-rays
- The only indication for skull X-rays is to evaluate for sinus disease.

Computerized Tomography (CT) Scans
- Excellent initial investigations for all cerebral lesions, particularly because it is quick and universally available.
- Excellent use in trauma, intracerebral hemorrhage, and shift of midline structures.
- Contrast enhancement is necessary for evaluation of stroke and neoplasms.
- Weaknesses of CT scanning: Fails to show infarcts for up to 24 h, unable to detect early stage subdural hematomas, lack of anatomic detail, fails to identify multiple sclerosis plaques, and detection of neoplasms requires contrast enhancement.
- If used with myelography, CT scanning may be helpful in spine disease or ruptured disks.
- May be a necessary test in patients who cannot undergo MRI scanning (e.g., claustrophobia, pacemaker, metallic stent, aneurysmal clips).

Magnetic Resonance Imaging (MRI)
- Gives excellent anatomic detail and shows virtually all structural diseases.
- Diffusion weighting image (DWI) is extremely valuable to identify early stroke signs.
- Apparent diffusion coefficient (ADC) maps may show restricted diffusion (e.g., stroke).
- Perfusion imaging is helpful in demonstrating area at risk in stroke (ischemic penumbra).
- Gradient echo is helpful for hemorrhage, both old and new.
- T2 weighting shows edema and white-matter lesions well.
- FLAIR sequences are useful for evaluation of multiple sclerosis.
- Contrast enhancement with gadolinium will show neoplasms and enhanced meninges.
- A superb noninvasive test for spinal cord disease or herniated disks in cervical or lumbar region.

Imaging of the Cerebral Circulation
- Magnetic resonance angiography (MRA) is the initial imaging of choice; 2-D time of flight shows extracranial circulation (vertebrals and carotid bifurcations); 3-D time of flight demonstrates intracranial circulation; contrast-enhanced studies will show aortic arch and aortic branches.
- CT angiography (CTA) with reconstructed views also demonstrates cervical and intracranial circulation well; better than MRA for detecting cerebral aneurysms.
- Magnetic resonance venogram (MRV) may be performed to evaluate suspected venous sinus occlusion.
- Carotid duplex ultrasound is noninvasive method of identifying carotid stenosis; widely used but accuracy is very technician-dependent; less useful for posterior circulation.
- A combination of MRI, CTA, and carotid Doppler usually accurately determines the degree of carotid stenosis; otherwise, catheter angiogram may be necessary.
- Transcranial Doppler may be helpful in identifying intracranial stenosis or occlusion; also used to identify cerebral emboli as there is an audible signal that can be imaged as well; however, highly technician-dependent.
- Catheter angiography is still considered by some to be the "gold standard" for identifying arterial stenosis and aneurysms; carries a 1% risk of stroke as a complication; generally necessary only to determine the degree of extracranial carotid artery stenosis in preparation for endarterectomy or stenting; however, accuracy of MRA, CTA, and Doppler ultrasound is usually sufficient such that catheter angiogram is needed only where uncertainty remains; may be necessary to identify arteriovenous malformations.

10. Lumbar Puncture & CSF Analysis

- Lumbar puncture is performed less commonly today, as imaging and other noninvasive diagnostic tests are readily available. However, it is still necessary to diagnose meningitis and suspected subarachnoid hemorrhage if imaging results are inconclusive.
  - There are no absolute contraindications to lumbar puncture if the information is required to diagnose meningitis.
  - Relative contraindications include bleeding tendency (platelets below 20,000 or elevated INR), intracranial mass lesion (especially in posterior fossa), and skin infections at site of puncture.

Procedure
- Perform in a sterile field at the interspace between L4-5 or L5-S1 (a line between the iliac crests roughly corresponds to the L3-4 interspace).
- Positioning is important! Arrange the patient with knees flexed up to the chest as much as possible and chin tilted down to the chest with back flexed.
- Spinous processes should be palpated; when interspace is located and marked, administer local anesthesia to the area.
- The spinal needle should be directed slightly cephalad until a palpable pop is felt, which marks the dura-arachnoid; at that point, CSF should begin to flow.
- It is best to ask patient to rest supine for several hours after the lumbar puncture (although its value is unproven).
- Opening pressure measurement with manometer.
  - Pressure measurement is generally not necessary unless pseudotumor cerebri or low spinal fluid pressure syndrome is suspected.
  - Normal pressure is 100–200 mm H_2O (will fluctuate with respirations and Valsalva).
  - If opening pressure is high, replace the stylus and allow pressure to come down slightly before taking samples.
  - Closing pressure may be measured and is usually slightly lower than opening pressure.
- Difficult lumbar punctures may result in traumatic taps resulting in bloody CSF drainage. These may occur as a result of movement with an uncooperative or delirious patient, severe obesity and poor landmarks, or osteoarthritis and calcification of the ligamentum flavum.
- Other complications include sudden, severe radicular pain from nerve root irritation and post-spinal tap headaches in about 20% of patients.

Typical CSF Samples for Analysis
- Cell count: Normally there are 0–6 WBCs. RBCs are normally absent unless a traumatic tap occurred, subarachnoid or cerebral hemorrhage is present, or herpes simplex encephalitis is present.
- Glucose: Normally 50–60 mg/dL or 50–60% of serum glucose.
- Protein: Normally 50–60 mg/dL. If traumatic tap, allow 1 additional mg/dL for each 1000 RBCs.
- Cultures and sensitivity.

Special CSF Tests for Analysis
- Cytology: If meningeal cancer suspected. Several studies may be necessary to identify tumor cells
- Special cultures, including TB, fungal, and viral cultures.
- PCR evaluation to detect DNA may be necessary for a variety of viral and bacterial infections.
- Markers for specific neurological disorders (e.g., 14-3-3 protein for Creutzfeldt-Jakob disease).
- Oligoclonal banding and quantitative IgG in patients with multiple sclerosis or subacute sclerosing panencephalitis.
- ACE levels in suspected sarcoidosis.
- Unusual antibodies may be present in paraneoplastic conditions (e.g., anti-yo antibodies in paraneoplastic cerebellar degeneration).

Common CSF Abnormalities in Infections
- Elevated WBC count: Mild-to-moderate elevations in viral infections with mostly lymphocytes (which may begin as predominance of PMNs); higher counts tend to occur in bacterial infections with at least 90% PMNs
  - In addition to infection, other causes of pleocytosis (increased WBCs) include acute exacerbation of multiple sclerosis, sarcoidosis, cerebral neoplasm, cerebral infarction, NSAID or IVIG use, cerebral vasculitis, meningeal cancer, seizures, and migraine.
- Glucose is typically decreased (less than half of serum value) in bacterial infections, TB, fungal infections, and meningeal cancer but is normal in viral meningitis.
- Protein is typically moderately elevated in bacterial infections but normal in viral meningitis.
- Gram's stain and cultures are usually positive in untreated bacterial meningitis.

10. Lumbar Puncture & CSF Analysis

Common CSF Abnormalities in Subarachnoid Hemorrhage

- Fluid is either bloody or xanthochromic (pink- or yellow-tinged) and under high pressure (nonhemorrhagic causes of xanthochromia include hyperbilirubinemia and excessively elevated CSF protein >350 mg/dL).
- If traumatic tap is suspected, spin CSF in centrifuge and observe supernatant; if the supernatant is xanthochromic, then subarachnoid hemorrhage is suspected since oxyhemoglobin has been released; if clear, then likely traumatic tap.
- Bilirubin appears in the CSF by the third day and lasts 2 wk; if subarachnoid hemorrhage is suspected, CSF may be positive for 2 wk.
- Protein is usually moderately elevated.
  - Other causes of elevated CSF protein include tumors, myxedema, acute exacerbation of multiple sclerosis, diabetes mellitus, polyneuropathy, Guillain-Barré syndrome, and spinal block due to cancer, lymphoma, or infection.
- Glucose may be low or normal.

11. EEG & Evoked Potentials

Electroencephalography (EEG)

• EEG is dynamic test of electrical activity of the brain.
  –Performed by placing electrodes on the scalp, amplifying the activity, and displaying it on a monitor or paper.
  –Brain waves are summations of excitatory and inhibitory potentials that are projected through the reticular nucleus of the thalamus to the cerebral cortex. Spikes represent polarization shifts of groups of neurons in the cortex. Slow waves may emanate from the white matter and represent a disruption of neural pathways.
  –The normal EEG changes in the early years of life but becomes standardized during adolescence.
  –EEG should be evaluated in cases of suspected seizure or any altered state of consciousness.
  –The normal EEG includes findings in the wake and sleeping state.
  –In the awake, resting state, most of the record will demonstrate alpha activity (8–12 Hz rhythm). Beta activity (greater then 13 Hz) may be seen in the frontal areas. A small amount of theta activity (4–8 Hz) may be present. Delta activity (1–4 Hz) is always abnormal in an awake patient.
  –Before and during sleep, drowsiness is often exhibited by low-voltage fast activity. Theta activity is seen in stages 2 and 3 of sleep. Stage 4 sleep is predominantly delta activity. REM sleep is characterized by low-voltage fast activity.

Abnormal EEG patterns

• Generalized spike-and-wave discharges are seen in primary generalized seizures. Three per second spike-and-wave patterns are characteristic of absence seizures.
• Focal spike or spike-and-wave discharges may be seen in partial epilepsies.
• Induction of sleep or sleep-deprived states may be necessary to detect complex-partial seizure patterns. Repeat studies are often necessary.
• Synchronous discharges may occur in active seizures.
• Periodic discharges may occur in nonconvulsive status epilepticus.
• Generalized slowing (mostly delta and theta activity) is seen in metabolic encephalopathy, postictal states, and dementias. May also be seen with whole brain infections (e.g., encephalitis) or anoxia.
• Focal slowing is seen in focal lesions, such as tumors, strokes, AV malformations, and brain abscesses.
• Medium voltage fast activity (greater than 12 Hz) may be seen with minor tranquilizer use (e.g., benzodiazepines, barbiturates).
• Focal temporal lobe discharges occur in herpes simplex encephalitis.
• Periodic epileptiform discharges occur in Creutztfeldt-Jakob disease.
• Periodic lateralized epileptiform discharges occur in strokes.
• Burst-suppression patterns occur in severe anoxic encephalopathy.
• Triphasic wave forms occur in hepatic and other encephalopathies.
• Electrocerebral silence is seen with brain death.

Closed Circuit Television (CCTV) Monitoring

• CCTV monitoring is a modality in which patients are evaluated continuously by simultaneous EEG and videotaping for a day to a week or longer.
  –Allows clinicians to evaluate the relationship of brain activity to physical seizure activity (e.g., convulsions, staring spells).
  –Often used to distinguish psychogenic seizures from epilepsy or syncope from seizures.
  –Also used to localize the site of seizure discharge in preparation for epilepsy surgery.

Evoked Potentials

• Evoked potentials are potentials recorded from the cortex following stimulation of various sensory pathways of the nervous system.
  –Visual evoked potentials (VEPs): Electrodes placed over the occipital lobes will record visual stimuli (usually alternating checkerboard flash patterns are used in each eye as the stimulus); latency is normally 100 msec; delayed latency may occur with optic neuritis or multiple sclerosis.
  –Brainstem-auditory evoked response potentials (BAERs): Electrodes placed over the auditory cortex will record a variety of cerebral potentials following auditory signals (usually a click); can help distinguish lesions of the auditory nerve (e.g., acoustic neuroma) from brainstem disease (e.g., stroke) by the shape and distribution of the evoked potentials.
  –Somatosensory evoked potentials (SSEPs): Electrodes placed on peripheral nerves (e.g., sural nerve in foot, median nerve in the hand) will record stimulation of peripheral nerves; commonly used during spinal surgery to determine if there has been an interruption in nerve or spinal transmission.

12. EMG & Nerve Conduction Studies

• Electromyography (EMG) and nerve conduction studies are used to evaluate for abnormal function of the PNS.

Electromyography (EMG)

• EMG primarily evaluates the function of the motor unit. It is performed by inserting a needle into muscles and recording the amplified potentials on an oscilloscope.
  – Anterior horn cell diseases, nerve root disease, and occasionally nerve diseases cause fasciculations (a spontaneous contraction of the motor unit).
  – Lesions of the motor unit (e.g., ALS, nerve root disease, neuropathies) lead to reduced numbers of functional motor units and result in reduced number of recruited motor units upon muscle contraction.
  – Neurogenic diseases produce denervation potentials, such as fibrillations and positive waves (spontaneous contraction of muscle cells).
  – In muscle diseases, EMG shows abundant, small-amplitude potentials due to random muscle cell damage that crosses the boundaries of the motor units. However, the number of motor units recruited are normal
  – It may take 2–3 wk for the EMG to become positive after nerve damage.

Nerve Conduction Studies

• Nerve conduction studies evaluate for neuropathies by measuring the rate of conduction of a stimulus through a peripheral nerve.
  – Nerve conduction velocities become abnormal or slowed primarily with demyelinating neuropathies (e.g., peripheral neuropathies, Guillain-Barré syndrome, chronic immune demyelinating polyneuropathy, mononeuritis multiplex) and with axonal neuropathies (e.g., alcoholic, uremic, idiopathic small fiber, and AIDS-related neuropathies).
  – Distal latencies measures nerve conduction across the neuromuscular junction to evaluate for compressive neuropathies such as carpal tunnel syndrome.
  – Repetitive nerve stimulation testing is also performed to evaluate disorders of the neuromuscular junction (e.g., in myasthenia gravis, a 3–5 Hz stimulation of the nerve will show decremental decreases of neuromuscular transmission; in Lambert-Eaton myasthenic syndrome, rapid stimulation of nerves at 30 Hz will result in an increased size of response).

Headache

Section 2

JON BRILLMAN, MD, FRCPI

13. Migraine Headache

Etiology/Pathophysiology

- An extremely common syndrome associated with headache and neurologic symptoms
- An inflammatory disorder of the brain and intracranial vasculature resulting in hyperreactivity of cerebral vessels
- Pathogenesis is complex; the aura has been associated with intra- and extracranial vasoconstriction and slow spread of excitation across the brain (referred to as "spreading depression"); the headache phase may be associated with vasodilatation of intra- and extracranial vessels and inflammation caused by activation of the trigeminal nerves and the blood vessels it supplies
- Increased binding of serotonin to platelets
- Classified as migraine with aura (formerly known as classical migraine), migraine without aura (formerly known as common migraine), and complex migraine
- An inherited disorder, likely autosomal dominant
- Up to 20% of the population experiences migraines

Differential Dx

- Stroke
- TIA
- Tension headache
- Sinus headache
- Subarachnoid hemorrhage
- Transient global amnesia

Presentation/Signs & Symptoms

- A prodrome of mood changes, insomnia, or nausea may occur with or without an associated aura
- Aura may be present, which is generally associated with visual phenomena (e.g., scotoma, flashes of light, zigzag lines, fortification spectra)
- The headache may be severe or mild, usually throbbing, and usually unilateral (migraines without aura are generalized)
- Numbness of extremities
- Photo- and/or phonophobia
- Nausea and vomiting

Diagnostic Evaluation

- History and neurologic examination
- CT scan or MRI of brain to rule out stroke or hemorrhage
- Lumbar puncture if subarachnoid hemorrhage is suspected

Treatment/Management

- Identify and avoid triggers (e.g., red wine, cheese, chocolate, alcohol, nitrates)
- Acute attacks may respond to rest in a dark, quiet room, triptan medications (oral, nasal, or parenteral), ergotamines, NSAIDs or other analgesics, corticosteroids, isometheptene, sedatives, and antiemetics
- For patients who experience more than one migraine per week, prophylactic medications should be considered, including β-blockers and/or calcium-channel blockers, tricyclic antidepressants, SSRIs, or anticonvulsants

Prognosis/Complications

- Headaches generally diminish with age but may persist
- May exacerbate with pregnancy, alcohol, or stress

14. Complicated Migraine

Etiology/Pathophysiology

- A migraine variant associated with a variety of neurologic signs and symptoms
- Associated with alterations in intracranial circulation and brain inflammation
- Stroke-like symptoms are probably caused by vasoconstriction of intracranial vessels
- Episodes of confusion and vomiting are likely related to excessive autonomic activity
- Ophthalmoplegic migraine often occurs after headache and may be due to compression of the third cranial nerve by a dilated, distended posterior cerebral artery
- Homonymous hemianopsia without headache in young persons represents vasoconstriction of the posterior cerebral artery
- Basilar migraine is seen commonly in young women due to ischemia to the brainstem
- Retinal ischemia may occur from vasoconstriction of retinal arterioles
- Some cases may lead to cerebral infarction, which is often associated with smoking and oral contraceptive use

Differential Dx

- Partial seizure
- TIA or cerebral infarction
- Drug intoxication
- Encephalitis
- Benign positional vertigo
- Gastroenteritis
- Central retinal artery occlusion
- Transient global amnesia
- Demyelinating disease

Presentation/Signs & Symptoms

- Headache may or may not occur
- Homonymous hemianopsia
- Hemiparesis
- Focal paresthesias in extremities
- Amnesia
- Confusion
- Aphasia
- Nausea and vomiting
- Third nerve palsy with pupillary involvement (ophthalmoplegic migraine)
- Transient monocular blindness ("retinal migraine")
- Fortification spectra in vision ("zigzag" lines and patterns)
- Vertigo occurs in basilar migraines

Diagnostic Evaluation

- History and neurologic examination
- MRI or CT scan of the brain to exclude structural lesion; may show microvascular infarcts
- MRA or CTA to exclude vascular disease
- Carotid duplex may be indicated to evaluate the extracranial circulation
- CSF exam is rarely necessary but may show mild pleocytosis
- Catheter angiogram is rarely necessary but may rule out an aneurysm in cases of ophthalmoplegic migraine

Treatment/Management

- There is no proven treatment for acute attacks
- Daily use of NSAIDs or aspirin may prevent attacks
- In contrast to simple migraine headaches, triptans are contraindicated in complicated migraines because they exacerbate the vasoconstriction
- Tricylic antidepressants, SSRIs, β-blockers, or calcium channel blockers may be prophylactic
- Avoid triggers (e.g., stress, chocolate, cheese, red wine)

Prognosis/Complications

- Prognosis is generally favorable with treatment
- Attacks tend to disappear with age

15. Cluster Headache

Etiology/Pathophysiology

- A severe, unilateral upper facial headache that is pulsatile in nature
- Occurs in clusters of about 2 wk, then may disappear for months or years
- Follows a seasonal (fall and spring) and periodic pattern
- Pathophysiology involves paroxysmal dilatation of facial arteries
- May be associated with autonomic dysfunction (e.g., rhinorrhea, lacrimation, Horner's syndrome)
- Seen mostly in males
- Smoking and alcohol may exacerbate the headaches
- No inheritance pattern

Differential Dx

- Migraine
- Sinus headache
- Tension headache
- Trigeminal neuralgia
- Subarachnoid hemorrhage
- Chronic paroxysmal hemicrania
- Temporal arteritis

Presentation/Signs & Symptoms

- Intense pulsatile pain over or around one eye
- May radiate into the entire side of the head and face
- Frequently nocturnal
- Lasts 20–45 min
- May be associated with nausea
- Horner's syndrome (ptosis, miosis, and anhidrosis) may occur
- Swelling of the eyelid may rarely occur

Diagnostic Evaluation

- History and neurologic evaluation
- Imaging (CT scan or MRI of the brain) is indicated to evaluate for cerebral pathology (e.g., retro-orbital lesions)
- Sinus X-rays
- Lumbar puncture with CSF analysis is indicated if infection or intracranial bleed is suspected

Treatment/Management

- Sumatriptan is the treatment of choice and may be administered by IV, oral, or nasal routes
- Avoid tobacco and alcohol
- Supplemental O_2 (6 L/min) may abort attacks
- A 2-wk tapering course of steroids is often used
- A 2-wk course of lithium may also be used (measure lithium levels weekly)

Prognosis/Complications

- Favorable prognosis with treatment and avoidance of precipitating factors

16. Tension Headache

Etiology/Pathophysiology

- Likely the most common cause of headache in the U.S.
- Due to muscle tension resulting in ischemia to the scalp and facial muscles
- May be associated with bruxism (grinding of teeth), emotional upset, intense concentration, and sleep deprivation

Differential Dx

- Headache due to mass lesion
- Migraine
- Sinus headache
- Functional or psychiatric headache
- Temporal arteritis
- Cervical arthritis

Presentation/Signs & Symptoms

- Headache is pressure in type in "hat-band" distribution or occipital region
- Aching, nonpulsatile sensation
- Bioccipital or bitemporal facial aching may be present
- Headache tends to occur late in the day
- Generally lasts 1–2 h
- Grinding of teeth may be noted in the history
- Neurologic examination is normal

Diagnostic Evaluation

- In most cases, history and neurologic examination is sufficient
- Brain imaging may be useful, primarily to relieve patient anxiety

Treatment/Management

- Most cases respond to analgesics and/or relaxation exercises
- A regular program of physical activity and exercise is beneficial
- Muscle relaxants, tranquilizers, or SSRIs may be used in severe cases

Prognosis/Complications

- Prognosis often depends on psychiatric comorbidities and ability to handle stress
- May be lifelong

17. Sinus Headache & Myofacial Pain Syndrome

Etiology/Pathophysiology

- Pain or pressure in the face due to inflamed sinuses or spasm of the muscles of mastication
- Pain is dull and boring, exacerbated by changes in barometric pressure (e.g., flying in airplane)
- Sinus pain occurs in the frontal areas of face due to pressure on sinus walls
    - May be associated with active or chronic sinus infections
- Myofacial pain results from spasm of muscles of mastication due to grimacing, bruxism (grinding of teeth), and anxiety
    - Related to tension headaches

Differential Dx

- Migraine
- Tension headache
- Trigeminal neuralgia
- Intracranial neoplasms
- Cluster headache
- Chronic paroxysmal hemicrania
- Temporal arteritis
- Dentalgia

Presentation/Signs & Symptoms

- Facial pain
- Swelling and tenderness over the sinuses occurs in sinusitis
- Pain with chewing
- Deviation of jaw upon mouth opening occurs in myofacial spasms
- Tenderness over temporomandibular joint

Diagnostic Evaluation

- Complete history and physical examination
- Sinus films including plain X-rays, CT scan, or MRI
- X-ray or CT scan of the temporomandibular joint
- Brain imaging may be indicated
- ESR should be measured in elderly patients to rule out temporal arteritis
- Panoramic X-ray of teeth and gingiva

Treatment/Management

- Sinusitis may respond to decongestants and antibiotics
- Analgesics
- Mouth guard may be helpful for bruxism
- Physical therapy with facial massage may occasionally be useful
- Surgical intervention may be indicated for temporomandibular joint disease
- Muscle relaxants are often used for myofacial pain
- ENT referral may be indicated in severe or recurrent cases

Prognosis/Complications

- Sinusitis tends to be chronic with frequent exacerbations
- Myofacial pain syndrome usually responds to aggressive therapy

18. Headache Due to Analgesic Overuse

Etiology/Pathophysiology

- Daily headaches that are related to excessive use of analgesic medications or triptans
- Overuse is defined as multiple daily dosing of medication beyond the prescribed dose
- Likely the major cause for chronic daily headache
- Related to fluctuating blood levels of analgesics (as blood levels of analgesics decline, headache increases)
- Related to psychoneuroses and drug dependency

Differential Dx

- Migraine headache
- Tension headache
- Psychogenic headache
- Drug-seeking behavior

Presentation/Signs & Symptoms

- Analgesic overuse headache: A pressure-type headache that waxes and wanes but is persistent to some degree
- Triptan overuse headache: A pulsatile headache similar to migraines

Diagnostic Evaluation

- Careful history and neurologic examination
  - Index of suspicion should be high if headache occurs daily
- Imaging (CT scan or MRI of the brain) is indicated in most cases of initial onset of headache
  - Repeat imaging may be necessary if the character of the headache changes
- Psychiatric evaluation may be helpful

Treatment/Management

- Patient education and proper administration of medication is imperative
- A "drying out" period may be necessary with hospitalization and administration of corticosteroids with gradual withdrawal of the offending medication
- Psychiatric consultation may be necessary, including substance abuse counseling

Prognosis/Complications

- Prognosis depends heavily on psychiatric factors
- Poor prognosis if personality disorders and drug dependency exist

19. Pseudotumor Cerebri

Etiology/Pathophysiology

- A disorder of brain swelling seen primarily in women of childbearing years
- Results in extracellular brain edema of unknown etiology
- Findings are attributable to increased intracranial pressure, including headache, papilledema, and sixth nerve palsy
- Seen almost exclusively in young females of childbearing years with menstrual irregularities
- Patients are often obese
- Pregnancy is a risk factor
- Rarely seen in males
- May be associated with a variety of endocrinopathies (e.g., Addison's disease, hypoparathyroidism), steroid withdrawal, excessive vitamin A intake (including Retin-A), or tetracyclines
- Possibly related to increased venous sinus pressure and reduced absorption of CSF at the arachnoid villi
- As opposed to hydrocephalus, the ventricles are not enlarged

Differential Dx

- Headache due to a mass lesion
- Tension headache
- Migraine
- Pseudopapilledema

Presentation/Signs & Symptoms

- Headache, primarily in the mornings, is the most common complaint
- Nausea
- Tinnitus
- Transient obscurations of vision (brief blurring of vision upon change of position)
- Visual blurring
- Cranial nerve VI palsy resulting in diplopia
- Papilledema

Diagnostic Evaluation

- History and neurologic examination to confirm signs of increased intracranial pressure in the absence of neurologic findings
- CT scan or MRI of the brain to rule out mass lesions or hydrocephalus
- Magnetic resonance venography to exclude venous sinus occlusion
- Lumbar puncture with opening and closing pressure measurements and CSF analysis
    - Imaging must be completed initially to rule out a mass lesion; however, in contrast to cases of increased intracranial pressure due to a mass lesion, brain herniation is of little concern with pseudotumor cerebri
    - All CSF constituents are normal
    - CSF pressure is greater than 200 mm H_2O
- Visual field testing and acuity measurement should be done in an ophthalmology lab to accurately assess subtle visual field deficits

Treatment/Management

- Treatment involves long-term reduction of increased intracranial pressure
- Discontinue offending agents (e.g., tetracycline, Retin-A)
- Weight reduction
- Acetazolamide or furosemide are used to decrease the production of CSF
- Lumboperitoneal shunt may be necessary if diuretics and weight reduction are ineffective
- Optic nerve fenestration to reduce pressure on the optic nerve is necessary in rare cases to avoid permanent visual loss
- Repeated CSF drainage may be done via lumbar punctures but is uncomfortable and generally ineffective

Prognosis/Complications

- Often a self-limited disorder that resolves with therapy within a year or two
- Visual loss is the most feared complication; occurs in about 5% of cases
- Visual field testing must be followed regularly

20. Low Spinal Fluid Pressure Headache

Etiology/Pathophysiology

- Hypoliquorrhea is an occipital and nuchal headache caused by traction on the pain-sensitive structures at the base of the brain as a result of low spinal fluid pressure
- Follows a lumbar puncture in about 20% of cases; continued fluid leak occurs into paraspinal tissues may occur following a lumbar puncture resulting in low spinal fluid pressure
- Repeated attempts at lumbar puncture is a risk factor
- Either viral infections or minor trauma may precipitate "spontaneous" low spinal fluid pressure syndrome in the absence of lumbar punctures

Differential Dx

- Cervical arthritis
- Tension headache
- Migraine
- Brain tumor
- Meningitis
- Subarachnoid hemorrhage

Presentation/Signs & Symptoms

- Occipital headache that is exacerbated by orthostasis (erect posture) and improves with recumbancy
- Severe neck pain, which is also exacerbated by orthostasis and improves with recumbancy
- Meningismus may be present
- Nausea and vomiting
- Sixth nerve palsy (inability to abduct eye)

Diagnostic Evaluation

- History and neurologic evaluation
- MRI typically demonstrates thickened meninges and excessive dural enhancement thought to be due to venous stasis
- CSF pressure is extremely low, typically less than 60 mm H_2O and often not measurable
- Mild lymphocytic pleocytosis and elevated protein is often present
- Spontaneous low spinal fluid pressure syndrome may be associated with persistent CSF leak, which may be identified by radionuclide studies

Treatment/Management

- Most cases resolve within 2-3 d with bed rest alone
- Increasing fluid intake is of uncertain value
- Analgesic medications may provide symptomatic relief
- Caffeine ingestion (oral or IV) has been shown to improve the headache
- Autologous "blood patch" in region of the presumed leak is beneficial in 80% of cases (inject blood into the epidural space, which may seal the leak)

Prognosis/Complications

- Post-lumbar puncture headache is benign and generally clears up after a few days of rest and treatment
- Prognosis of spontaneous low spinal fluid pressure syndrome is less certain but often responds to blood patch

21. Temporal Arteritis

Etiology/Pathophysiology

- An inflammatory condition of unknown cause that affects all layers of the walls of extracranial arteries, most often the temporal artery
  - Involves medium-sized arteries all over body but mostly in the distribution of extracranial carotid arteries
  - Commonly involves the posterior choroidal arteries that supply the optic disc
  - Arteries become thickened and obstructed, resulting in ischemic nodules on the scalp
  - Lymphocytic infiltrates in the arterial wall, including giant cells, may be demonstrated on microscopy
- The classic picture of temporal arteritis is an elderly patient complaining of a new onset of unilateral headache, visual loss, and myalgias
- Untreated cases may lead to blindness
- One of three entities that are a part of giant cell arteritis: Polymyalgia rheumatica, aortic arch syndrome, and temporal arteritis
- Primarily occurs in patients over age 60
- Females > males
- Often associated with proximal aching in extremities (polymyalgia rheumatica)

Differential Dx

- Migraine
- Tension headache
- Cervical arthritis
- Intracranial mass headache
- Myofacial pain syndrome
- Cluster headache
- Central retinal artery occlusion
- Anterior ischemic optic neuropathy
- Fibromyalgia

Presentation/Signs & Symptoms

- Headache is pusatile or pressure-like; may be localized to the inflamed artery or generalized
- Jaw claudication with chewing
- Arthralgias/myalgias
- Low-grade fever
- Malaise
- Weight loss
- Transient monocular blindness or sudden loss of vision occurs in 25–50% of patients
- If vision is lost in one eye, there is greater than 50% likelihood of visual loss in the other eye within 1 mo
- Ophthalmoparesis
- Pale optic disc
- Indurated temporal artery

Diagnostic Evaluation

- History and physical exam
- CBC may show leukocytosis and/or normocytic anemia
- Elevated ESR (often greater than 80 mm/h) occurs in 90% of patients
  - Patients who are taking corticosteroids or aspirin may have a falsely lowered ESR
- C-reactive protein is also elevated
- Biopsy of the superficial temporal artery is diagnostic
  - A long segment of the artery is required because of skip areas
  - If negative but temporal arteritis is still suspected, a biopsy of the contralateral temporal artery should be done

Treatment/Management

- Responds well to high-dose corticosteroids
  - Prednisone should be started in high doses (80 mg/d) in suspected cases, even before biopsy is performed
  - Results of the biopsy will not be altered by steroid therapy for up to 2 wk
  - Steroid-sparing attempts with alternate-day steroid dosing is not recommended
  - Dosage of steroids should be gradually lowered when the patient becomes asymptomatic and ESR falls to about 25 mm/h
- Cyclophosphamide and methotrexate may be used in steroid-intolerant patients
- Treatment should be maintained for 18 mo to 2 y

Prognosis/Complications

- The disease is generally adequately controlled with steroids; corticosteroids are usually tolerated well despite the advanced age of patients
- Relapse is common if steroids are discontinued too soon
- Untreated, it can lead to blindness: 50% of patients will lose sight in one or both eyes
- Once blindness occurs, it is often permanent; however, if therapy is started after unilateral vision loss, the other eye is protected
- ESR and C-reactive protein may be used to monitor response to treatment
- After 2 y of treatment, relapses are rare (less than 20% of cases)

22. Headache Due to Subarachnoid Hemorrhage

Etiology/Pathophysiology

- See also *Subarachnoid Hemorrhage* entry in the Cerebrovascular Disease section
- Nontraumatic subarachnoid hemorrhage is most commonly due to rupture of cerebral aneurysm into the subarachnoid space
- Larger aneurysms are more prone to rupture
- Rupture may occur spontaneously but often occurs with valsalva, coughing, or straining
- Rupture usually occurs at ages 50–70
- 30% of cases are multiple

Differential Dx

- Migraine
- Exertional headache
- Coital headache
- Tension headache
- Low spinal fluid pressure headache
- Peri-mesencephalic hemorrhage due to venous bleeding

Presentation/Signs & Symptoms

- Sudden onset of explosive headache, often termed "the worst headache of my life"
- 50% of patients have alteration of consciousness, including seizures
- Meningismus (stiff neck) is usually present
- Subhyaloid hemorrhages can be seen on surfaces of the retinas
- Stroke or coma may occur secondary to vasospasm

Diagnostic Evaluation

- Characteristic history and physical examination
- 95% of CT scans show subarachnoid and/or intraventricular blood
- Lumbar puncture is indicated if the diagnosis is uncertain
  - Xanthochromia (pink CSF) begins 2–4 h after bleed begins, representing presence of oxyhemoglobin
  - Opening pressure is elevated
  - Elevated RBCs are present initially; protein becomes elevated after several days
  - The abnormal CSF color may remain for 3 wk due to the presence of bilirubin released by lysis of RBCs
- CT angiogram is indicated to evaluate the intracranial vasculature; an excellent modality to detect aneurysms
  - MRA may miss small aneurysms
- Angiography is still the gold standard to diagnose aneurysms; however, may be negative in 20% of cases

Treatment/Management

- Initial treatment of SAH includes rest, BP control, sedation, and control of intracranial pressure
  - Hypertension may cause an aneurysm to rebleed; hypotension may cause cerebral ischemia
  - Control of intracranial pressure may include head elevation, mannitol, hyperventilation (pCO_2 30–35), CSF drainage, placement of an intraventricular drain
- Seizure prophylaxis with IV phenytoin
- Ruptured aneurysms should be surgically clipped emergently if the patient is stable
  - Control BP carefully; maintain fluid volume with normal saline or Ringer's lactate
  - Patients should be sedated
  - Nimotopine should be administered to prevent secondary vasospasm and stroke
  - Endovascular coiling is reserved for inaccessible aneurysms

Prognosis/Complications

- SAH carries an overall 50% mortality
- 25% of patients have permanent impairment
- Prognosis is improved if patient is not in coma
- Rerupture may occur within the first 3 wk
  - Rerupture of an untreated aneurysm occurs at a rate of about 3% per year, cumulatively
  - Clipped aneurysm rarely, if ever, rebleeds
- 20% of patients have a normal angiogram
  - Prognosis is better in these patients
  - Repeat angiogram recommended after 1 wk
- Secondary vasospasm is a feared complication that occurs in 30% of cases
  - May result in stroke or coma
  - Usually occurs after the third day
  - Prognosis worsens if vasospasm occurs
- Communicating hydrocephalus may occur in 12–24 h and may requires shunt or draining
- SIADH may occur with hyponatremia

23. Intracranial Mass Headache

Etiology/Pathophysiology

- These headaches occur due to traction on the pain-sensitive structures in the skull (e.g., dura at base of the brain, vascular sinuses, irritation of cranial and cervical nerves) by a mass lesion
- Mass lesions include primary or metastatic tumors, brain abscess, epidural or subdural hematoma, venous or sinus occlusion, trauma with edema, encephalitis, subdural empyema, and arteriovenous malformation

Differential Dx

- Migraine
- Tension headache
- Cluster headache
- Temporal arteritis
- Cervical arthritis
- Chronic daily headache
- Chronic paroxysmal hemicrania
- Analgesic overuse headache
- Pseudotumor cerebri

Presentation/Signs & Symptoms

- Unilateral headache, pressure in type
- Positional headache exacerbated by valsalva (e.g., cough) and relieved by upright posture
- Worse in the morning
- Associated with seizures, fever, focal neurologic signs or visual disturbances
- Posterior fossa lesions irritate the upper cervical nerves and refer pain to the back of head and neck
- Frontal or middle fossa lesions irritate cranial nerve V and refer pain to the face
- Nausea and vomiting
- Hiccups

Diagnostic Evaluation

- History and neurological exam
- CT or MRI of the brain with and without contrast
- MRV if venous sinus disease or pseudotumor cerebri is suspected
- Lumbar puncture with CSF analysis to exclude infection should only be done after mass lesion is excluded by imaging

Treatment/Management

- Relieve elevated intracranial pressure by head elevation, mild hyperventilation (e.g., $pCO_2 = 35$ mm Hg), mannitol or furosemide administration, and/or surgical drainage
- Neurosurgical intervention may be indicated for internal decompression or total extirpation of a mass
- Corticosteroids may be administered to decrease edema
- Thrombolysis or anticoagulants for venous sinus occlusion
- Analgesics for pain control

Prognosis/Complications

- Prognosis depends entirely on the nature of underlying condition and ability to remove the mass or structural lesion from pain-sensitive intracranial structures

24. Trigeminal Neuralgia

Etiology/Pathophysiology

- Also known as tic douloureux
- A form of intense facial pain due to irritation of trigeminal nerve
- Most cases are idiopathic
- The pathogenesis is obscure but may be related to compression of the trigeminal nerve by vascular structures in the posterior fossa (e.g., a dilated ectatic basilar artery, neuroma, artery, or vein)
- Lancinating, sudden pain in the face within the distribution of the trigeminal nerve and lasting just seconds
  - V_2 is most commonly affected followed by V_3; V_1 involvement is rare
- Occurs primarily in older patients but may be seen in young patients with multiple sclerosis due to a brainstem plaque in the trigeminal nucleus

Differential Dx

- Post-herpetic neuralgia
- Tolosa-Hunt syndrome
- Cluster headache
- Myofacial pain syndrome
- Facial migraine
- Dentalgia
- Sinus headache

Presentation/Signs & Symptoms

- Sudden, severe, unilateral, lancinating pain in face in the distribution of the trigeminal nerve (not below the angle of the jaw or behind the ear)
- Trigger zones are common (e.g., touching face or tooth with eating utensils, shaving, applying makeup)
- Episodes of pain, although brief, may be multiple
- Treatment may decrease the intensity of pain but may result in increased length of pain
- Rarely nocturnal

Diagnostic Evaluation

- History and neurologic examination
- MRI of brain is indicated to exclude structural lesions and multiple sclerosis
- MRA is often useful to demonstrate cerebral vessels that may compress the trigeminal nerve
- Sinus X-rays to exclude sinusitis
- Panoramic views of the teeth are rarely necessary

Treatment/Management

- 80% of cases are controlled with medication alone
- Carbmazepine is generally the treatment of choice
- Phenytoin or gabapentin may be used
- As most patients are elderly, low dosages are often used as these patients often have a low tolerance to medications
- Stereotactic injection of the trigeminal nerve with phenol or radiofrequency destruction of the nerve may improve symptoms but will leave the face numb
- Posterior fossa microvascular decompression should be reserved for intractable cases; best used when compression of the trigeminal nerve is demonstrated by imaging

Prognosis/Complications

- 80% of cases are controlled with medication alone
- 90% of patients respond to medical or surgical therapy
- Spontaneous remissions occur in 25% of cases
- Relapse rate is about 1% per year

Cerebrovascular Disease

JON BRILLMAN, MD, FRCPI

25. Transient Ischemic Attack

Etiology/Pathophysiology

- A transient (less than 1 h) episode of neurologic dysfunction secondary to reduced blood flow to the brain
- TIAs serve as warnings for subsequent stroke
  - Most strokes occur within 90 days of a TIA
  - Risk of subsequent stroke following an untreated TIA is 8–10% per year
- Etiologies are identical to those of ischemic stroke
  - Thrombosis of an atherosclerotic vessel
  - Lacunar infarcts (usually secondary to long-standing hypertension or diabetes)
  - Carotid stenosis
  - Cardioemboli (e.g., secondary to atrial fibrillation)
  - Arterial dissections
- The specific syndrome is related to the area of ischemia
  - Carotid ischemia results in anterior circulation TIA, causing dysfunction of the cerebral hemispheres and eyes
  - Vertebrobasilar ischemia results in posterior circulation TIA, causing dysfunction of the structures of the posterior fossa (e.g., cerebellum, brainstem), portions of the temporal lobe, and the occipital lobe

Differential Dx

- Syncope (consciousness is *not* lost during a TIA)
- Stroke
- Partial seizure
- Hypoglycemia
- Transient global amnesia
- Migraine
- Drug or alcohol intoxication
- Acute compression neuropathy (e.g., radial nerve palsy)
- Positional vertigo (may mimic posterior circulation TIA)
- Panic attack or hyperventilation syndrome

Presentation/Signs & Symptoms

- Anterior circulation TIA: Focal paresis, paresthesias, loss of sensation (arm, leg, and/or face
  - Transient monocular blindness less common; entire visual field or upper or lower half
  - Speech disturbance if dominant hemisphere involved
- Posterior circulation TIA
  - Cerebellar: Ataxia, dysarthria, dizziness
  - Brainstem: Diplopia, dysarthria, ataxia, quadraparesis, drop attacks, nystagmus, ophthalmoparesis
  - Occipital lobe dysfunction: Binocular visual loss or blurring
  - Dysmetria (abnormal finger-to-nose test)
- Babinski sign may occur with either anterior or posterior TIA

Diagnostic Evaluation

- History and neurologic examination (TIA is rarely associated with loss of consciousness)
- Initial laboratory studies include CBC, platelets, glucose, lipid profile, homocysteine level, and C-reactive protein (coagulation profile is indicated in younger patients)
- CT scan is used to rule out hemorrhage, tumor, or infarct
  - Acute infarct will not show up on CT for at least 24 h
- MRI with diffusion weighting will reveal acute infarct within minutes of occurrence
- Echocardiogram to evaluate cardiac sources of emboli
  - Transesophageal echo is more accurate than transthoracic
- CTA or MRA are used to evaluate for extra- and intracranial arterial stenosis or occlusion
- Carotid and vertebral Doppler studies also used to evaluate for arterial stenosis or occlusion
- Catheter angiogram is now used less frequently

Treatment/Management

- Risk factor modification includes smoking cessation, weight loss and exercise, blood pressure control, appropriate management of diabetes
- All suspected TIA patients should be placed on antiplatelet therapy, including aspirin, clopidogrel (Plavix), or dipyridamole/aspirin (Aggrenox)
- Statin therapy for hyperlipidemia
- Anticoagulation may be indicated in patients with a cardiac source of emboli
- Carotid endarterctomy is indicated if >70% stenosis is present in the appropriate carotid artery
- Endovascular carotid stenting is less invasive than carotid endarterectomy and may be indicated in high-risk patients if carotid endarterectomy cannot be performed

Prognosis/Complications

- TIA is a warning sign for subsequent stroke
  - The likelihood of stroke is 8–10% per year for the first year following a TIA and then about 5% per year over the next 5 y
  - The greatest risk of subsequent stroke is during the initial 90 d following a TIA
- Risk of stroke can be reduced by 50% if all risk factors are addressed

26. Acute Stroke Syndromes

Etiology/Pathophysiology

- Acute stroke is most commonly due to embolic occlusion of an intracranial artery (carotid occlusion, cardiac embolus, or primary thrombotic process) or small vessel occlusion
- Reversibly ischemic brain tissue (penumbra) occurs within the first few hours of stroke onset
- Reversibility is a function of the level of blood flow and the time it is maintained
    - The lower the blood flow, the less time it can be tolerated before irreversible changes occur
    - The shorter the time interval since onset, the greater the likelihood of reversibility
    - Multiple factors may modify reversibility, including age, existing collaterals, location of occlusion, blood pressure, and intermittent occlusion
    - In some cases, reversibility may persist up to 6–12 h from stroke onset
    - There have been reports of reversibility after up to 24 h with basilar artery occlusions

Differential Dx

- Seizure
- Migraine
- Hypoglycemia
- Hemorrhage
- Bell's palsy
- Conversion/hysteria
- Subdural hematoma
- Syncope
- Multiple sclerosis

Presentation/Signs & Symptoms

- MCA syndrome
    - Left MCA: Aphasia, right side weakness, left gaze preference, and somnolence
    - Right MCA: Dysarthria, left sided weakness, right gaze preference, left neglect, and denial of deficit
- ACA syndrome
    - Left ACA: Expressive speech difficulty, right sided weakness (leg and foot more than proximal arm), relative sparing of hand and face, grasp response
    - Right ACA: Dysarthria, left sided weakness (more in leg and foot)
- Basilar syndrome: Vertigo, diplopia, ocular bobbing, absent horizontal eye movements, unilateral hemiparesis, quadriparesis or hemiplegias, coma

Diagnostic Evaluation

- CT scan of the brain without contrast is indicated emergently to rule out hemorrhage
    - May reveal early ischemic changes, including hyperdense MCA sign (bright arterial signal), hypodensity (ischemic area), sulcal effacement, loss of insular ribbon, and obscuration of the basal ganglia
- CTA or MRA of intracranial and extracranial arteries to evaluate for occlusion
- Transcranial Doppler ultrasound may be used to supplement angiographic data of the intracranial circulation
- CT or MR perfusion scan to evaluate for the area of underperfused brain (ischemic penumbra)
- MRI with diffusion imaging is used to reveal the area of brain that is likely irreversibly damaged; positive within a few hours (earlier than CT changes)
- Initial laboratory studies should include chemistries, glucose, CBC with platelets, and PT/INR

Treatment/Management

- IV thrombolysis with tPA if within 3 h of stroke onset and if CT without hemorrhage or extensive hypodensity; NIHSS 4 or greater and not rapidly improving; BP <180/110; no recent stroke or MI; no history of intracranial tumor, bleed, or AVM; no recent head trauma; and no recent surgery or punctures at noncompressible sites
- If 3–6 h from stroke onset, consider intra-arterial tPA if CT without hemorrhage or extensive hypodensity, NIHSS at least 10, and (if imaging available) evidence of large vessel occlusion
- Other possible treatments: combined IV/intra-arterial thrombolysis, emergent angioplasty or stenting
- No proven effective neuroprotective agents
- After thrombolysis, follow BP closely to maintain BP <180/110 and avoid antiplatelet agents and anticoagulants for 24 h

Prognosis/Complications

- Patients should be monitored closely in an ICU setting for 24 h; neurosurgical consult and follow-up CT scan at 24 h
- Frequent neuro checks; emergent CT scan for any neurologic changes
- Intracerebral hemorrhage is the major complication of thrombolytics
    - Hemorrhage with clinical deterioration occurs in 6% of patients after IV tPA, up to 10% after intra-arterial thrombolysis
    - For patients treated with IV tPA within 3 h of onset of symptoms, recovery to normal or near normal status occurs in 40%
    - For patients treated with intra-arterial thrombolysis within 6 h of onset of symptoms, recovery to independent status occurs in 40%
- Outcomes are best for MCA occlusion

27. Ischemic Stroke

Etiology/Pathophysiology

- Ischemic strokes constitute >80% of cases of stroke
- Thrombotic strokes are most common; due to arteriosclerosis
    - May be intracranial (usually occlusive) or extracranial (carotid or vertebral stenosis or occlusion)
    - Pathophysiology of atherosclerotic ischemic stroke involves artery-to-artery emboli, thrombosis, or perfusion deficits (e.g., complete occlusions of carotid artery, insufficient cardiac output)
    - May be associated with hypercoagulable states (e.g., antiphospholipid antibody syndrome, factor V Leiden, pregnancy, oral contraceptive use)
- Lacunar infarcts (see *Lacunar Stroke*) account for 30% of ischemic strokes: Small vessel occlusions producing limited neurologic deficits
- Cardioembolic infarcts (see *Embolic Stroke*) account for 25%
- Arterial dissections (see *Arterial Dissection*) are the most common cause of ischemic stroke in patients <50 years old; mostly due to trauma
- The vascular territory involved determines associated neurologic deficits
    - Carotid ischemia results in anterior circulation stroke causing dysfunction of the cerebral hemispheres and eyes
    - Vertebrobasilar ischemia results in posterior circulation stroke causing dysfunction of the structures of the posterior fossa (e.g., cerebellum, brainstem), portions of the temporal lobe, and the occipital lobe

Differential Dx

- Complicated migraine
- Hemorrhagic strokes
- Seizures
- Metabolic encephalopathy
- Syncope
- Positional vertigo
- Multiple sclerosis
- Conversion hysteria
- Neoplasm
- Mononeuropathy (e.g., radial nerve palsy)
- Bell's palsy

Presentation/Signs & Symptoms

- Depends on distribution (see *TIA*)
- Anterior circulation stroke: Focal weakness, sensory alterations, or aphasia
- Posterior circulation stroke syndromes often have a more complex presentation
    - Thalamic infarct: Sensory, thalamic pain
    - Midbrain tegmentum infarct: Contralateral tremor, ophthalmoparesis
    - Midbrain peduncle infarct: Contralateral hemiparesis, ophthalmoparesis
    - Pontine infarct: Gaze plegia, pinpoint pupils, internuclear ophthalmoplegia, quadriparesis, "locked-in" state, coma
    - Occipital: Homonymous hemianopsia
    - Lateral medulla: Crossed sensory, ataxia, dysarthria, hoarseness, Horner's
    - Medial: Tongue deviation, hemiparesis

Diagnostic Evaluation

- History and neurologic examination
- Initial laboratory studies include CBC, platelets, glucose, lipid profile, homocysteine level, and C-reactive protein (coagulation profile is indicated in younger patients)
- Head CT without contrast to evaluate for hemorrhage, tumor, and infarct; however, acute infarcts will not show up on CT for at least 24 h
- MRI with diffusion weighting will reveal acute infarct within minutes of occurrence
- Echocardiogram to evaluate for cardiac source (TEE is much more accurate than TTE to detect cardiac emboli)
- CTA or MRA to evaluate for extra- and intracranial arterial stenosis or occlusion
- Carotid and vertebral Doppler studies are also used to evaluate for arterial stenosis or occlusion
- Catheter angiogram is now used less frequently, but is still the gold standard to diagnose arterial stenosis

Treatment/Management

- Acute therapy includes stabilization of glucose and BP (lower BP only when >220/115), as it may be necessary to maintain cerebral perfusion (do not lower SBP below 180)
- Thrombolytic therapy may be indicated if within 3 h of symptom onset (note 6% hemorrhage risk)
    - Intra-arterial thrombolytic therapy is reserved for MCA or basilar occlusion in tertiary care centers
- Anticoagulation with heparin is often used but there is no evidence that it improves outcomes
- Secondary prevention includes antiplatelets (aspirin, clopidogrel, dipyridamole/aspirin), statin therapy for hyperlipidemia, and BP control
- If cardiogenic source is found (e.g., A-fib), chronic anticoagulation with warfarin is indicated
- Carotid endarterectomy (or percutaneous stenting) is indicated in cases of carotid stenosis >70% in the symptomatic artery

Prognosis/Complications

- 20% immediate mortality
- 70% have some degree of disability
- Recurrence of stroke occurs at a rate of about 10% per year in untreated patients
    - Antiplatelet agents reduce the rate of stroke recurrence by 20%
    - Statins and blood pressure control (especially ACE inhibitors) reduce recurrence by 30%
    - Further risk factor modification includes smoking cessation, weight loss and exercise, and appropriate management of diabetes
- 50–70% of patients regain independence
- Up to 80% regain the ability to walk
- Nearly 50% of stroke victims will eventually die of MI
- Physical, occupational, and speech therapy are extremely helpful and should be started early

28. Embolic Stroke

Etiology/Pathophysiology

- Embolic strokes account for about 25% of all ischemic strokes
- Most common etiology is cardiac emboli that lodge in a cerebral vessel
  - Frequently embolize from the left atrium or the left-sided heart valves
  - The ascending aorta may be source of atheromatous emboli
- Non-valvular A-fib is a common cause
  - Patients with untreated, sustained A-fib have a 6% per year incidence of stroke
- Patients with a patent foramen ovale (with right to left shunt) may be at increased risk for stroke
  - The pathophysiology is unclear
  - Hypotheses include paradoxical emboli from the deep venous system in the extremities, atrial vulnerability (intermittent A-fib), or in situ clots on the atrial septum
  - Atrial septal aneurysm with patent foramen ovale may increase risk of stroke
- Bacterial endocarditis with resulting septic emboli results in stroke in about 10% of patients with endocarditis
- Embolic events may rarely occur from artery-to-artery (originate from the aorta and carotid arteries and embolize to smaller intracerebral arteries)

Differential Dx

- Ischemic infarcts secondary to carotid or vertebrobasilar atherosclerosis
- Lacunar infarct
- Seizure
- Migraine
- Intracerebral hemorrhage
- Tumor

Presentation/Signs & Symptoms

- Sudden onset of monoparesis (arm *or* leg involvement) or hemiparesis (arm *and* leg involvement)
- Sensory symptoms restricted to one extremity
- Posterior circulation is involved in about 20% of cases, most commonly resulting in ataxia, diplopia, visual blurring, or dysarthria
- Seizures may occur
- Signs of the underlying etiology may be present (e.g., heart murmur in valvular disease, irregular heartbeat in atrial fibrillation, fever in endocarditis)

Diagnostic Evaluation

- The general workup is similar to other ischemic strokes (see *Ischemic Stroke*)
- ECG should be evaluated to rule out atrial fibrillation
- Consider blood cultures if a murmur or valvular vegetation is present
- TTE is used to screen for cardiac sources of emboli but only identifies 15% of embolic sources
- TEE is much more accurate than TTE but is invasive
  - Will identify left atrial clots, appendage clots, or aortic atheroma
  - Bubble study is necessary to evaluate for patent foramen ovale

Treatment/Management

- General approach to stroke patients (see *Ischemic Stroke*)
- Anticoagulation is indicated in nearly all patients with chronic, nonvalvular A-fib
  - Contraindications include lone A-fib in young patients, intolerance to coumadin, and significant risks of fall or bleeding
  - Begin with heparin (target PTT of 2½ times control) followed by coumadin (target INR 1.8–3.0)
- Aspirin is of little utility, but does confer some protection if coumadin cannot be used
- Treatment of a patent foramen ovale is uncertain; aspirin, warfarin, and endovascular or surgical closure are all considerations
- If blood cultures are positive, institute appropriate antibiotics
  - Anticoagulation is contraindicated in patients with endocarditis

Prognosis/Complications

- Embolic stroke may result in large infarction with hemorrhagic conversion, especially if anticoagulation has been started
- 20% of patients present with "malignant stroke" characterized by massive edema of a hemisphere and herniation; this syndrome carries a high mortality
- Seizures may occur
- Anticoagulation reduces the rate of stroke by 70%, but may result in bleeding (especially in the elderly)
- Physical and occupational therapy is an important adjunct of treatment

29. Lacunar Stroke

Etiology/Pathophysiology

- Lacunar strokes are small infarcts (less than 1.0 cm) in the distribution of small-caliber arteries that have no collateral circulation (e.g., lenticulostriates and penetrating vessels of the brainstem and cerebellum)
- Occur in the basal ganglia/internal capsule area, brainstem, and cerebellum
- Account for 30% of all ischemic strokes
- Occur primarily due to long-standing hypertensive disease
    - The underlying pathology involves lipohyalinosis, which damages the intima of small caliber arteries/arterioles, causing intimal swelling and occlusion of blood flow
- Infarcts are generally small and may be silent
    - Multiple small infarcts may be asymptomatic and eventually lead to dementia (multi-infarct dementia)
    - Binswanger's disease is the most common type of multi-infarct dementia: Coalescent infarcts in the centrum semiovale (in white matter of brain) result in a syndrome of dementia and gait disturbances

Differential Dx

- Ischemic infarct secondary to large-vessel occlusion
- Hypertensive bleed (often occurs in the same site as lacunar infarct)
- Embolic stroke
- Multiple sclerosis (in younger patients)
- Sensory seizures
- Other causes of dementia
    - Alzheimer's disease
    - Pick's disease
    - Lewy body dementia
- Migraine

Presentation/Signs & Symptoms

- Pure motor hemiparesis
- Ataxic hemiparesis (clumsiness of extremities)
- Dysarthria
- Pure sensory symptoms may occur if thalamus is involved
- Gait apraxia and dementia occurs with Binswanger's disease
- Pseudobulbar features may include spontaneous crying, dysarthria, dysphagia, and primitive reflexes (e.g., snouting, increased jaw jerk)

Diagnostic Evaluation

- History and neurologic examination
- Initial laboratory studies include CBC, platelets, glucose, lipid profile, homocysteine level, and C-reactive protein (coagulation profile is indicated in younger patients)
- CT reveals small rounded or oval infarcts in the area of the basal ganglia, centrum semiovale, brainstem, or cerebellum
    - Asymptomatic disease is frequently incidentally observed on imaging studies
- MRI with or without DWI is more sensitive than CT scan
- Echocardiogram to evaluate for cardiac source
- Evaluate for coexistent large vessel disease (i.e., intra- or extracranial arterial stenosis or occlusion) by CTA, MRA, carotid and vertebral Doppler studies, or angiogram

Treatment/Management

- BP control is by far the most important aspect of treatment
    - Target of 120/80
- Antiplatelet medication (aspirin, clopidogrel, and/or dipyridamole/aspirin) should be instituted in all patients unless contraindicated
- Cessation of smoking
- Statin therapy in patients with hyperlipidemia
- Antidementia agents (e.g., donepezil, memantine) are often used for multi-infarct dementia but have not been proven to be useful
- Physical therapy for gait training in affected patients

Prognosis/Complications

- Prognosis is generally favorable, as these strokes are small
- Untreated lacunar infarcts may lead to larger ischemic strokes, intracerebral hemorrhage, or dementia

30. Intracerebral Hemorrhage

Etiology/Pathophysiology

- Bleeding into the parenchyma of the brain tissue
- Most commonly associated with hypertension
    - Long-standing hypertension leads to lipohyalinosis, which results in fragility of deep, penetrating arterioles, and Charcot-Bouchard aneurysms, which may rupture
    - Hypertensive bleeds occur in the basal ganglia (60%), thalamus (20%), pons (10%), and cerebellum (10%)
- Other causes include trauma (most common cause in younger patients), arteriovenous malformations, cavernous angiomas, anticoagulation and antithrombolytic therapy, CNS vasculitis, leukemia, acquired thrombocytopenia and DIC, moyamoya disease, cocaine and amphetamine use
    - Amyloid angiopathy is the most common cause of hemorrhage in the elderly; results in lobar hemorrhage

Differential Dx

- Ischemic infarct
- Migraine
- Subarachnoid hemorrhage
- Cerebral neoplasm
- Positional vertigo (may be confused with cerebellar hemorrhage)

Presentation/Signs & Symptoms

- Acute onset of headache
- Focal paresis
- Gaze deviation to the side of lesion (20% may be to the contralateral side)
- Nausea/vomiting
- Results in significant hypertension
- Thalamic hemorrhage results in sensory alteration and numbness of an extremity
- Cerebellar hemorrhage results in gaze deviation away from lesion, occipital headache, vomiting, ipsilateral ataxia
- Pons hemorrhage results in pinpoint pupils, quadriplegia, stupor, and coma
- Lobar hemorrhage causes symptoms related to the involved lobe (e.g., confusion in frontal hemorrhage, hemianopsia in occipital hemorrhage)

Diagnostic Evaluation

- History and neurologic examination
- Initial laboratory studies should include a coagulation profile
- Head CT scan or MRI without contrast (gradient echo) will show hyperdensity in the brain parenchyma
- Angiography may identify arteriovenous malformations but are rarely seen after bleeds

Treatment/Management

- Management of BP is essential to prevent expansion of hemorrhage
    - If pressure exceeds 220/120, administer labetalol, nitropaste, or nifedipine to lower BP to 150/90
    - Nitroprusside drip is indicated if SBP exceeds 250 mm Hg
- Trials have not shown surgical intervention to be of value in basal ganglia bleeds unless transtentorial herniation is imminent
- Cerebellar hemorrhages may require surgical intervention for removal of blood if patient shows signs of brainstem compression or tonsillar herniation
- Physical therapy is beneficial
- Factor VII administration has been shown to restrict bleeding in one trial

Prognosis/Complications

- Complications include seizures, SIADH, hydrocephalus, and focal neurologic deficits
- Prognosis is favorable if herniation does not occur, often with less resultant disability than ischemic infarcts
- Interventricular extension of hemorrhage is a poor prognostic sign
- Recurrence is unusual if BP is adequately controlled
- Recurrence is more likely in amyloid angiopathy

31. Subarachnoid Hemorrhage

Etiology/Pathophysiology

- The most common cause of SAH is trauma
- Of nontraumatic subarachnoid hemorrhages, at least 80% are due to ruptured intracerebral saccular ("berry") aneurysms in the region of the circle of Willis
  – Incidence is uncertain but estimated to be about 5% of the population
  – Most likely result from a defect of the media of an intracerebral artery at birth with progressive enlargement secondary to atherosclerosis
  – About 5% rupture, causing sudden increase of intracranial pressure
  – Most ruptures occur between 40 and 70 years of age
  – 25% occur in the anterior cerebral or communicating arteries, 25% in the internal carotid or posterior communicating arteries, 25% in the middle cerebral circulation, and 25% in the posterior circulation
  – 15–20% are multiple
  – 10–15% are familial
- Arteriovenous malformations are a less common cause of SAH
- Mycotic aneurysms are rare; seen in endocarditis due to metastasis of infected material from heart valves to the intracerebral arterial wall
- Also rarely caused by arterial dissection or vasculitis
- Peri-mesencephalic hemorrhage may be due to venous bleeding, with favorable prognosis

Differential Dx

- Migraine
- Cluster headache
- Tension headache
- Syncope
- Seizure
- Hypertensive intracerebral hemorrhage
- Meningitis

Presentation/Signs & Symptoms

- Sudden, explosive onset of headache ("worst headache of my life")
- Syncope or seizures may occur
- Altered mental status, including stupor or coma, occurs in 50% of cases
- Meningismus is often present
- Papilledema
- Photophobia
- Subhyaloid hemorrhages are visible on the surface of retina
- Hemi- or quadriparesis
- Nausea/vomiting
- Third cranial nerve paresis (may include mydriasis) may occur with unruptured internal carotid-posterior communicating aneurysm

Diagnostic Evaluation

- Head CT without contrast will reveal subarachnoid blood in 95% of cases
- If clinical suspicion persists despite negative CT, lumbar puncture is indicated to look for xanthochromia (pink-yellow fluid), which will be present in all cases within 2–10 h of an SAH
  – The CSF will remain discolored for 3 wk due to oxyhemoglobin and bilirubin
  – Other findings include elevated RBC count, increased opening pressure, elevated protein, and leukocytosis
- CTA and MRA are the gold standard to identify a ruptured aneurysm
- Catheter angiogram is indicated if the diagnosis is still in doubt; may be negative in 20% of cases due to spasm or clotting

Treatment/Management

- Initial treatment: Rest, BP control (HTN may cause an aneurysm to rebleed; hypotension may cause cerebral ischemia), sedation, and control of intracranial pressure (head elevation, mannitol, hyperventilation, CSF drainage, or placement of intraventricular drain)
- Seizure prophylaxis with IV phenytoin
- Asymptomatic aneurysms may be followed by serial CTAs if smaller than 10 mm
- Larger unruptured aneurysms may be treated with endovascular coil placement
- Ruptured aneurysms should be surgically clipped emergently if the patient is stable
  – Control BP carefully and maintain fluid volume with normal saline or Ringer's lactate
  – Patients should be sedated
  – Nimotopine should be administered to prevent secondary vasospasm and stroke

Prognosis/Complications

- Overall 50% mortality; 25% of patients have permanent impairment
- Prognosis is improved if patient is not in coma
- Rerupture may occur within the first 3 wk
  – Rerupture of untreated aneurysm occurs at a rate of about 3% per year, cumulatively
  – Clipped aneurysm rarely, if ever, rebleeds
- Coiling of aneurysms is a promising treatment but cure rates are unknown
- 20% of patients have a normal angiogram
  – Prognosis is better in these patients
  – Repeat angiogram recommended after 1 wk
- Secondary vasospasm is a feared complication that occurs in 30% of cases (usually after day 3) and may result in stroke or coma
- Communicating hydrocephalus may occur in 12–24 h and may require shunt or draining
- SIADH may occur with hyponatremia

32. Arterial Dissection

Etiology/Pathophysiology

- Arterial dissection occurs when tearing of an artery results in dissection of blood into the arterial wall, causing occlusion of the vessel with subsequent clot formation and embolic infarction
    - Occasionally, complete occlusion of the vessel results in hypoperfusion and infarction
- As opposed to aortic dissections with rupture, dissections of smaller vessels more commonly result in occlusion of the vessel and infarction
- Dissection is a common cause of stroke in young persons
    - Almost always occur secondary to trauma; athletic injury, whiplash-type injuries, and chiropractic manipulation are most common
    - Nontraumatic, spontaneous dissections may be seen in patients with migraines, fibromuscular dysplasia, Marfan's, and Ehlers-Danlos
- Involved arteries include the carotid artery (via compression against the transverse process of C2 vertebra) and the vertebral arteries in the v1 segment (at the bifurcation of the subclavian artery), the v3 segment (as it courses dorsally behind the atlas), or the v2 segment (in the transverse foramen of the cervical vertebrae)
- Arterial rupture may rarely occur secondary to the creation and rupture of a false lumen due to dissections through the media and adventitia

Differential Dx

- Migraine
- Ischemic stroke
- Cluster headache
- Idiopathic Horner's syndrome

Presentation/Signs & Symptoms

- Presents with the typical signs and symptoms of a TIA or stroke
- Neck or facial pain occurs with or without an associated stroke
- Horner's syndrome may occur
- Lingual paresis
- Tinnitus

Diagnostic Evaluation

- CT and MRI with "dissection protocol" (axial views) are diagnostic, revealing blood in the arterial wall
- CTA or MRA is used to identify the pattern of dissection, occlusion, or fibromuscular dysplasia
- Carotid duplex may be helpful to identify carotid stenosis or occlusion
- Catheter angiography is rarely necessary but shows a "string sign" or flame-shaped tapers
- Complete occlusion may occasionally be present and visualized by any of these modalities

Treatment/Management

- Antiplatelet therapy (e.g., aspirin, clopidogrel) alone may be a sufficient treatment to prevent subsequent stroke
- Anticoagulant therapy (e.g., coumadin) is commonly used but has not been proven to be better than antiplatelet agents
    - Most patients are started on anticoagulant therapy for 6 wk and then switched to aspirin or clopidogrel
- Surgical correction is not necessary but stenting may be useful if symptoms persist

Prognosis/Complications

- Prognosis is usually favorable
- Severe stroke occurs in only 10% of cases
- Recanalization of the dissected artery occurs within 6 mo in most cases
- Imaging with MRA and CTA should be repeated in several months to evaluate for recanalization
- Antiplatelet therapy should be continued indefinitely, regardless of whether recanalization occurs

33. Venous Stroke

Etiology/Pathophysiology

- An infarction of the brain that occurs secondary to stasis in venous system
- Usually associated with prothrombotic states (e.g., pregnancy and postpartum period, oral contraceptive usage, antiphospholipid antibody syndrome, factor V Leiden, protein C or S deficiency, sickle cell disease)
  –Occur due to coagulation of the slower-flowing venous blood
- Less common etiologies include trauma, dehydration, infection, cancer
  –Transverse sinus occlusion may result from middle ear infections
  –Cavernous sinus thrombosis may be secondary to facial or intracranial infections
- May occur in any of the cerebral sinuses or cortical veins
- The most common area of venous stroke is occlusion of the superior saggital sinus

Differential Dx

- Cerebral arteritis of puerperium
- Eclampsia of pregnancy
- Arterial stroke
- Pseudotumor cerebri
- Migraine
- Subarachnoid hemorrhage
- Intracerebral hemorrhage
- Intracranial arterial dissection

Presentation/Signs & Symptoms

- Headache
- Paraparesis (bilateral leg weakness) if the superior saggital sinus is involved
- Hemiparesis
- Stupor or coma
- Nausea/vomiting
- Seizures are more common in venous stroke than arterial stroke
- Papilledema
- Cavernous sinus occlusion results in swelling of the eye, ophthalmoparesis, chemosis, and mydriasis

Diagnostic Evaluation

- CT or MRI is used to identify areas of infarction and/or hemorrhage
- MRV should be used to identify venous occlusion; however, it is unreliable due to variations of venous anatomy
- Catheter venogram is indicated to evaluate the venous anatomy if thrombolytic therapy is being considered
- Hypercoagulable profile, including PT/PTT, factor V Leiden mutation, antiphospholipid antibody, lupus anticoagulant, antithrombin III

Treatment/Management

- Anticoagulants are the primary treatment, but must be used with great caution as there is a significant risk of secondary hemorrhage
- Hydration
- Thrombolytic therapy via transvenous catheterization is reserved primarily for some cases of superior saggital sinus thrombosis
- Antiplatelet agents (e.g., aspirin, clopidogrel) may be used but have not been proven to be beneficial
- Appropriate antibiotic treatment of infection

Prognosis/Complications

- Prognosis is often favorable with complete recovery in weeks
- Cavernous sinus thrombosis may be fatal, particularly if associated with infection

34. Cryptogenic Stroke

Etiology/Pathophysiology

- A stroke of uncertain etiology that occurs primarily in young patients
- Accounts for 25–35% of all strokes
- Occurs in younger patients without typical stroke risk factors
- There have been associations identified with migraine syndromes, patent foramen ovale, mitral annular calcification, mitral valve prolapse, aortic arch atheroma, valvular strands, nonbacterial thrombotic endocarditis, sympathomimetic use, and hypercoagulability
- Possible etiologies include artery-to-artery embolus from a nonstenotic plaque, intermittent A-fib, undefined hypercoagulable states, cardiac abnormalities of uncertain association, and patent foramen ovale
    - Note: A patent foramen ovale is found in 35–50% of patients with cryptogenic stroke; there is a 3-fold increase in incidence of cryptogenic stroke with presence of a patent foramen ovale and even greater incidence with presence of patent foramen ovale and atrial septal aneurysm

Differential Dx

- Migraine
- Seizure
- Cerebral hemorrhage
- Vasculitis
- Neoplasm
- Transient global amnesia
- Bell's palsy
- Hysterical conversion reaction

Presentation/Signs & Symptoms

- Acute onset of focal neurological deficit
- Syndromes are usually suggestive of embolic events with deficits attributable to intracranial arterial occlusion or branch occlusions
- Cortical signs (e.g., visual field deficits, aphasia, neglect, anosognosia, hemiparesis, hemisensory loss)
- Brainstem syndromes less common

Diagnostic Evaluation

- MRI and MRA to evaluate tissue damage and vascular occlusions
- TEE to evaluate for patent foramen ovale and cardiac sources of emboli
- Hypercoagulable battery includes anticardiolipid antibody, lupus anticoagulant, factor V Leiden mutation, and prothrombin gene variant

Treatment/Management

- Antiplatelet agents are most commonly used to prevent further incidence of stroke
- In some cases, anticoagulation might be indicated, particularly if intermittent A-fib is suspected
- Treatment of stroke associated with antiphospholipid antibodies is unclear; recent evidence suggests coumadin may not be superior to aspirin
- Management of patients with cryptogenic stroke with associated patent foramen ovale is also uncertain; options include antiplatelet agents, anticoagulants, or endovascular closure of the patent foramen ovale

Prognosis/Complications

- Stroke recurrence occurs in up to 20% of patients over 2 y
- Patent foramen ovale is associated with 1–2% per year rate of stroke recurrent; incidence increases to 4% per year in patients with a patent foramen ovale and atrial septal aneurysm
- No clear advantage to anticoagulation compared to antiplatelet therapy for stroke associated with antiphospholipid antibodies

Seizures

Section 4

JAMES P. VALERIANO, MD

35. Tonic-Clonic Seizures

Etiology/Pathophysiology

- Formerly called grand mal seizures, these generalized seizures are characterized by a possible aura, a loss of consciousness and posture, a tonic phase lasting 10–20 s, a slightly longer clonic phase, and postictal confusion or stupor, which may last hours
- May be genetic in origin
  - Usually characterized on EEG by a three per second spike-and-wave discharge
  - Will often occur early in the morning, often upon waking
  - Often preceded by myoclonic jerks
- Acquired cases are usually considered secondarily generalized seizures that begin as partial seizures
  - Etiologies include any type of focal brain lesion including stroke, brain tumor, head trauma, and CNS infection
  - Drug or alcohol withdrawal is also a common cause of these seizures
  - Metabolic disturbances predispose to these seizures (e.g., hyponatremia, uremia, hypocalcemia, hepatic failure)
- May occur at any age: Generalized seizures often have onset in infancy and begin before 2 y; in general, these seizures have a peak incidence before the age of 20 with a second peak that occurs after the age of 60

Differential Dx

- Syncope
- Convulsive syncope
- Psychogenic seizures
  - Anxiety attacks
  - Panic attacks

Presentation/Signs & Symptoms

- Usually begin with generalized tonic stiffening of all extremities in extension
  - Diaphragmatic contraction occurs, resulting in loud grunting sound as air is forcefully expelled from the chest
- After tonic phase, generalized clonic jerking occurs in all four extremities with the arms often drawn into a flexed position, usually lasting 30–90 s
  - Tongue biting and incontinence
- A postictal phase follows the event, usually with 10–30 min of confusion/disorientation
- There may also be postseizure focal neurologic signs, often referred to as Todd's phenomena (e.g., aphasia, hemiparesis, hemisensory loss)

Diagnostic Evaluation

- Diagnosis is best made from an accurate description of the event, usually by an observer; key historical information includes duration of the event, the tonic-clonic progression of the event, and the postictal confusional period
- EEG done in the postictal state will show generalized slowing, may show focal or generalized spikes; during the seizure, EEG may show epileptiform abnormality as focal spikes or generalized spike-and-wave discharges
- CT and MRI may reveal focal lesions
- Trauma patients with generalized tonic-clonic seizures will usually have suffered some physical trauma from the event (e.g., fractures, abrasions, contusions, lacerations)
- Laboratory evidence of generalized seizures usually includes an elevated CK level and elevated prolactin
- Chemistries and drug/alcohol levels should be measured
- CSF analysis if suspect infection or hemorrhage

Treatment/Management

- Multiple medications are effective
  - In patients with primary or genetic generalized seizures, valproate remains the drug of choice
  - In secondary generalized seizures, numerous medications may be equally effective, including phenytoin, phenobarbital, topiramate, lamotrigine, zonisamide, levetiracetam, and carbamazepine
- These antiepileptic agents are relatively equal in efficacy for generalized tonic-clonic seizures; they differ primarily in side effect profile, drug interactions, and general tolerability
- Avoidance of alcohol or drug ingestion in appropriate patients
- Correct metabolic disturbances if present (e.g., hyponatremia, uremia)
- Anticonvulsant levels, liver function studies, and CBC must be periodically monitored

Prognosis/Complications

- Patients with a first generalized tonic-clonic seizure are felt to have about a 1/3 risk of recurrence within 2 y; this risk can be further defined by EEG findings (i.e., an abnormal EEG increases the risk)
- These seizures generally respond well to medications and have a good prognosis
- Prognosis also depends on etiology of the seizures (i.e., patients with focal lesion causing secondary generalized seizures such as stroke or brain tumor are more likely to have recurrent seizures than those with idiopathic generalized seizures)
- Seizures due to alcohol or drug withdrawal may not require anticonvulsant therapy
- In most states, patients may not drive for 6 mo to 1 y after any seizure with loss of consciousness

36. Absence Seizures

Etiology/Pathophysiology

- Inherited seizure disorder in the category of primary generalized epilepsy
- May represent a multifactorial inherence pattern consistent with autosomal dominant inheritance with variable penetrance
- Seizures arise from recruitment of increased electrical activity from the reticular-cortical system, frontal cortex, and hippocampus with a synchronous discharge to all areas of the cortex
- Not usually associated with neurological abnormality on neuroimaging, physical examination, or cognitive testing
- Absence seizures are divided into childhood absence (usually begins around age 7) and juvenile absence (usually begins around ages 12–14
- Nearly 15% of affected patients have first-degree relatives with epilepsy
- Approximately 50% of the siblings (age 4–10) of patients with absence seizures have EEGs with generalized spike-and-wave discharges; however, less than 10% of them will experience seizures
- Atypical absence (Lennox-Gastaut syndrome) is an acquired seizure that often occurs in severely brain-injured patients: Involves a brief loss of awareness and is usually combined with multiple seizure types, including complex partial seizures, tonic seizures, atonic seizures, myoclonic seizures, and generalized tonic-clonic seizures

Differential Dx

- Atypical absence seizure
- Complex partial seizure
- Daydreaming

Presentation/Signs & Symptoms

- Simple absence seizures consist of a brief lapse of awareness (3–10 s); patients may be unaware of the episode
  - Usually no postictal phase (i.e., patient will recover consciousness immediately upon cessation of the seizure)
- Complex absence seizures may involve a loss of muscle tone, myoclonic components, or even tonic stiffening
- Complex absence tends to occur as the seizures become more prolonged, usually if lasting beyond 10 s
- Lennox-Gastaut syndrome: Associated with drop attacks, myoclonic jerks, and absence-type seizures

Diagnostic Evaluation

- Diagnosis is usually made with the help of observers; patients are usually unaware that they have had a lapse of awareness unless they are aware they have missed part of a conversation or other events have transpired during their brief loss of consciousness
- There is often a family history of seizures, particularly of other primary generalized epilepsies
- The hallmark of diagnosis is the EEG, which shows a generalized three per second spike-and-wave discharge
  - If this discharge lasts more than 3 s, then a clinical seizure has occurred and the patient at that time will have lost consciousness
  - Lennox-Gastaut syndrome has a typical EEG ("hypsarrhythmia") characterized by constant 1–2 per second spike-and-wave patterns
- Neuroimaging studies are normal in pure absence epilepsy

Treatment/Management

- Nearly 100% of all absence seizures (except Lennox-Gastaut) can be prevented with antiepileptic medications
- Ethosuximide is drug of choice and will control approximately 80% of patients with absence seizures
- Valproate is also very effective, controlling about 80% of patients with absence seizures; valproate has the added advantage of controlling generalized tonic-clonic seizures, which occur in 40–50% of patients with absence seizures
- Newer medications that may be effective include lamotrigine, topiramate, levetiracetam, zonisamide
- Carbamazepine and tiagabine should be avoided as they occasionally worsen absence seizures and precipitate absence status epilepticus
- Lennox-Gastaut is generally refractory to treatment and requires several antiepileptic agents

Prognosis/Complications

- Approximately 40% of patients with childhood absence will develop generalized tonic-clonic seizures, with a somewhat higher rate occurring in juvenile absence epilepsy
- The vast majority of patients with childhood absence will have cessation of their absence seizures by age 20
- Juvenile absence epilepsy often continues into adulthood, with about 30% of patients still suffering absence seizures at age 40
- Lennox-Gastaut, in contrast to absence epilepsy, has a poor prognosis in terms of seizure control and progressive mental deterioration

37. Partial Seizures

Etiology/Pathophysiology

- Partial seizures occur secondary to focal brain lesions, which produce electrical discharges that are limited in scope and manifestations
  - Specific manifestations depend on site of lesion (e.g., parietal lobe lesions causing marching paresthesias in the opposite extremities, temporal lobe lesions result in bizarre behaviors)
- Focal brain injuries include stroke, brain tumor, CNS infections, congenital malformations, arteriovenous malformations, and head trauma
- Onset at any age due to the acquired nature of this type of epilepsy
- Often begin in adulthood, most commonly due to cerebrovascular disease and neoplasms
- The most common cause in adolescents is head trauma or idiopathic
- Simple partial seizures are focal sensory or motor events without loss of consciousness
- Complex partial seizures involve brief episodes of alterations in consciousness, often with bizarre sensations or manifestations (e.g., dream-like states, automatisms, olfactory sensations, mouthing or swallowing movements); usually due to lesions in the temporal or portions of the frontal lobes
- All partial seizures may secondarily generalize into tonic-clonic seizures

Differential Dx

- Absence seizures
- TIA/stroke
- Migraine
- Psychogenic events
- Pseudoseizure
- Transient global amnesia

Presentation/Signs & Symptoms

- Simple partial seizures do not involve lapse of awareness
  - Subdivided by symptomatology, including focal motor seizures, focal sensory seizures, and seizures with psychic phenomena
  - Psychic phenomena include déjà vu or jamais vu, depersonalization, or sense of unreality
  - Often evolve to complex partial seizures
- Complex partial seizures usually involve a 30–90 s loss of awareness, followed by 1–5 min of postictal confusion
  - Automatisms = purposeless movements (picking at clothes); orobuccal movements (lip smacking/swallowing)

Diagnostic Evaluation

- Diagnosis often depends on interviews with observers who have experienced the events
  - With complex partial seizures, the patient is amnestic through the event and the observer will often describe a blank stare with minor automatisms
  - Simple partial seizures are usually described by the patient, who details focal jerking of an extremity, focal sensory phenomena usually on one side of the body or one extremity, or psychic phenomena such as déjà vu
- EEG will often show focal abnormalities, including focal slow or sharp wave discharges from the presumed site of seizure origination
- Repeated EEG monitoring may be necessary
- In uncertain cases, CCTV may be necessary to witness the events
- MRI may also be helpful to delineate focal lesions

Treatment/Management

- Treatment options include many medications, including phenytoin, carbamazepine, oxcarbazepine, phenobarbital, primidone, zonisamide, topiramate, lamotrigine, tiagabine, and levetiracetam
  - Choice of medications is usually based on potential side effects and potential epidemiological considerations (e.g., possibility of pregnancy, interactions with other drugs, age, gender)
  - Anticonvulsant levels, CBC, platelets, and LFTs must be periodically monitored
- If medications fail, other treatment options include evaluation for epilepsy surgery with removal of seizure focus or vagal nerve stimulators

Prognosis/Complications

- Simple partial and complex partial seizures have a very high recurrence rate; these types of seizures are often refractory to medications and combinations of medications
- Remission is possible, though it is difficult to calculate remission rates; those who are more likely to remit include patients who have had fewer seizures, patients who have responded almost immediately to medications, and those who have relatively normal EEGs
- Prognosis also depends on the etiology of the seizure disorder, with more severe injuries or insults resulting in more refractory epilepsy
- Surgical intervention will improve patient response to anticonvulsants in 50% of refractory cases

38. Myoclonic Seizures

Etiology/Pathophysiology

- Myoclonic seizures are events characterized by repetitive jerking of large muscle groups and have a wide range of etiologies
- Often seen in patients with diffuse cerebral conditions involving the cerebral gray matter, including lipid storage diseases, infections (e.g., Creutzfeldt-Jakob disease, SSPE)
- Also may be acquired in adulthood due to metabolic disorders, such as uremia, anoxia, hyperosmolar states, and rarely paraneoplastic syndromes
- Can also occur with progressive neurologic diseases, such as progressive myoclonic epilepsy with or without Lafora bodies
- Can be seen as a primary generalized epilepsy such as juvenile myoclonic epilepsy or absence epilepsy with myoclonic components
- Frequently occurs in neonates due to neurodegenerative conditions (e.g., gangliosidosis, particularly Tay-Sachs disease, Alpers' disease)
- Acquired forms can occur at any time of life

Differential Dx

- Tremors
- Myokymia
- Focal motor seizures
- Tics
- Tetany
- Benign myoclonic jerks of early sleep
- Exaggerated startle responses

Presentation/Signs & Symptoms

- Myoclonic jerks are brief clonic movements that may occur sporadically in different parts of the body, may be confined to one limb, or may occur in a more generalized fashion involving the axial musculature
- Multifocal myoclonus is seen most commonly in diffuse metabolic disorders such as anoxia or uremia
- Myoclonic seizures can evolve into tonic-clonic seizures, such as occurs in juvenile myoclonic epilepsy

Diagnostic Evaluation

- Clinical observation of brief myoclonic jerks or a description of these by a patient or observer
- EEG can be helpful with primary generalized epilepsy with myoclonic components, often showing a three per second polyspike-and-wave discharge
    - –EEG may also be helpful to rule out epileptic myoclonus if no EEG correlate to myoclonic jerks can be found
- Serum chemistries should be evaluated to exclude metabolic etiologies of myoclonus
- Imaging may be indicated if the cause cannot be determined

Treatment/Management

- Multiple medicines may be effective, with benzodiazepines often being the most effective for short-term control
- For primary generalized epilepsy with myoclonus, valproate tends to be the most effective drug; other possibilities include topiramate, lamotrigine, zonisamide, and levetiracetam
- Treatment of the underlying condition, including metabolic conditions, is often necessary to fully treat myoclonus

Prognosis/Complications

- Prognosis depends on the etiology of the myoclonus
- Prognosis is very poor if myoclonus is part of a generalized neurodegenerative condition
- If myoclonus is due to metabolic derangements (e.g., uremia), correction of the underlying condition often results in substantial improvement of the myoclonus
- Primary generalized epilepsies with myoclonus are often successfully treated with valproate

39. Status Epilepticus

Etiology/Pathophysiology

- A medical emergency that is defined as a single seizure lasting for more than 30 min or multiple seizures that occur without fully regaining consciousness between events
  - May be nonconvulsive, mimicking a psychiatric disturbance
- There are multiple etiologies: Anticonvulsant withdrawal or noncompliance (subtherapeutic drug level) is the most common cause
- Other causes include brain tumor, stroke, CNS infections, head trauma, febrile illnesses, alcohol withdrawal, metabolic disturbances, anoxia
- 50,000–150,000 cases in the U.S. per year
- Most common at extremes of age (children under age 5 and adults over age 60), but may occur at any age
- 10% of patients with epilepsy will present with status epilepticus
- 50% do not have a history of epilepsy

Differential Dx

- Seizure clusters
- Psychogenic status epilepticus
- Coma
- Psychiatric disturbances (e.g., catatonia)

Presentation/Signs & Symptoms

- Repetitive seizures, usually three or more
  - Tonic-clonic seizures are most common; other types of seizures are also possible
  - May be convulsive or nonconvulsive
- Convulsive status
  - Repetitive generalized tonic-clonic seizures
  - Cyanosis
  - Increased BP
  - Tachycardia
  - Muscle headache
- Nonconvulsive status
  - Confusional state may be due to absence status epilepticus or complex partial status epilepticus

Diagnostic Evaluation

- Clinical observation with seizure activity lasting greater than 30 min
- Initial laboratory studies include CBC, chemistries, blood culture, and toxicology screen
  - Convulsive status epilepticus may result in acidosis, elevated CK, myoglobinemia, and myoglobinuria
- Spinal fluid analysis if infection is suspected
- EEG documents ongoing seizure activity, even if clinical seizures have stopped; EEG is imperative to diagnose nonconvulsive status epilepticus

Treatment/Management

- Treatment of the seizure should be started before waiting for any of the diagnostic tests to return—eliminate seizure activity, then treat the underlying condition
- Thiamine should be administered in alcoholics, glucose if hypoglycemic, naloxone if drug overdose is possible
- Intubation may be necessary for respiratory depression
- Initial antiepileptic agents include lorazepam or diazepam, phenytoin or fosphenytoin, or phenobarbital
- Seizures that remain refractory to the above medications may be treated with propofol, pentobarbital, or versed
- Monitor anticonvulsant levels

Prognosis/Complications

- Prognosis is related to the underlying condition
- Death occurs in 2–3% of children and 7–10% of adults
- Morbidity/mortality worsen quickly with duration of seizure
- Mortality worse at extremes of age
- Prolonged seizures can lead to permanent brain damage
- Release of catecholamines during seizures may trigger fatal cardiac arrhythmias

40. Febrile Seizures

Etiology/Pathophysiology

- Generalized convulsions that occur during febrile episodes; not associated with brain infection
- Most common cause of seizures in childhood
- Occurs in 2–4% of all children, generally between 6 mo to 6 y of age (peak at 18 mo)
- Seizure activity is related to degree of temperature elevation and the child's threshold for seizure (based on developmental state of brain)
- There is controversy as to whether the rate of rise of fever is important
- There is a genetic predisposition; 10–20% have a positive family history (first-degree relative)
- Typically occurs on the first day of illness
- Associated with viral illnesses such as otitis media, pharyngitis, or gastroenteritis
- May follow administration of vaccines

Differential Dx

- Syncope
- Benign focal epilepsy of childhood
- Absence epilepsy
- Tonic-clonic epilepsy
- Lennox-Gastaut syndrome
- Meningitis
- Encephalitis
- Toxins (e.g., salicylates, theophylline, Shiga toxin, anticholinergics)
- Electrolyte disturbances (e.g., hypoglycemia, hypocalcemia)

Presentation/Signs & Symptoms

- Generally associated with rapidly rising fever
- Simple febrile seizure: Generalized tonic-clonic activity lasting less than 15 min with associated fever
- Complex febrile seizure (15%) characterized by focal seizure activity, seizure duration beyond 15 min, or multiple seizures within a 24-h period
- Complex features may occur, such as Todd's paralysis (focal weakness during the postictal period)

Diagnostic Evaluation

- History and physical exam are usually diagnostic (typical age range, no prior neurologic disease, no focal deficits on physical exam); examination should include a search for focus of infection (e.g., ears, throat, lungs, abdomen)
- If a site of infection is identified, brain imaging and EEG are generally unnecessary
- EEG should be done in cases of prolonged or repeated seizures
  - EEG during the event will show seizure activity
  - May be normal, slow, or epileptiform following seizures (therefore it is not helpful if the child is not seizing)
- Brain imaging is indicated if focal seizures occur (either CT or MRI)
- Lumbar puncture with CSF analysis is indicated if meningeal signs or coma ensues
- Transient hyperglycemia may accompany seizures

Treatment/Management

- Supplemental oxygen and antipyretics should be administered during seizures
- Anticonvulsant therapy is not necessary for a single seizure
- Antiepileptic drugs (e.g., rectal diazepam, phenobarbital, valproate) should be administered for repeated, prolonged, or complex seizures or if there is a strong family history of febrile seizures
- Treat underlying infections as necessary

Prognosis/Complications

- Solitary febrile seizures have a benign prognosis—do not result in brain damage, neurologic defects, mental retardation, or learning disorders
- Recurrent febrile seizures tend to occur if there is a positive family history or early age of onset
- Prophylactic rectal valium upon onset of illness can prevent future febrile seizures; however, antipyretic therapy may not prevent seizures
- 35% overall risk of recurrence; 25% risk of recurrence during the next 12 mo
- Slightly increased risk for epilepsy; risk increases 4-fold with prolonged seizures (longer than 1 min), complex seizures, or with family history of febrile seizures
- No evidence that treatment of febrile seizures with anticonvulsants prevents later-life epilepsy

Movement Disorders

SUSAN M. BASER, MD

Section 5

41. Parkinson's Disease

Etiology/Pathophysiology

- A common, progressive disorder characterized by impoverished movements, rigidity, and tremor
- Dementia occurs in up to 35% of cases
- Results from the loss of dopaminergic neurons in the substantia nigra and other CNS areas
- Most cases are idiopathic
- Other types of parkinsonism can be drug-induced, due to a postsynaptic blockade of dopamine receptors; usually caused by psychotropic or antidopaminergic agents
- Average age of onset is about 60 y
- A common disorder—affects 1% of Americans over age 50
- Men are slightly more often affected than women
- Autopsy shows Lewy bodies in the brainstem and basal ganglia

Differential Dx

- Drug-induced parkinsonism
- Diffuse Lewy Body disease
- Progressive supranuclear palsy
- Shy-Drager syndrome
- Essential tremor
- Wilson's disease
- Gait apraxia
- Corticobasal ganglionic degeneration
- Normal pressure hydrocephalus
- Poisonings (e.g., carbon monoxide, methanol, manganese)

Presentation/Signs & Symptoms

- Classic triad of tremor (resting "pill-rolling" tremor decreasing with movement), "cogwheel" rigidity, bradykinesia (slow initiation of movement)
- Positive symptoms include tremor, rigidity, and flexed posture
- Negative symptoms include loss of reflexes, bradykinesia, and freezing
- Masked facies
- Difficulties with activities of daily living (e.g., dressing, eating, writing)
- Subcortical dementia (in 50–70% of cases)
- Seborrhea (oily skin), excess salivation
- Unstable posture with flexion of trunk and extremities and shuffling gait
- Festinating gait (propulsive tendencies)

Diagnostic Evaluation

- History and physical examination generally diagnostic
- Clinical response to therapy with dopamine agonists strongly suggests Parkinson's disease
- No laboratory test or imaging is diagnostic
- Should exclude Wilson's disease in young patients (low serum ceruloplasmin, high urine copper, Kayser-Fleischer rings)
- MRI should be obtained if dementia is present

Treatment/Management

- Discontinue all drugs with Parkinson's effect (e.g., metoclopramide, phenothiazines, haloperidol)
- Early cases can be observed for a period of time if no significant functional impairment is present
- Treatment is aimed at increasing the levels of dopamine in the CNS
  - Dopamine agonists are initially used, including ropinirole and pramipexole
  - Eventually, patients require levodopa plus carbidopa combinations
  - With time, effects of levodopa wear off; entacapone may be tried
- Amantadine may be helpful for short periods of time; useful for dyskinesias
- Selegiline is of variable benefit
- Surgical intervention with subthalamic deep brain stimulation is beneficial in patients with intractable dyskinesia, tremor or rarely, rigidity

Prognosis/Complications

- Disease advances in all cases, but the degree of progression varies from patient to patient
- Medications have prominent side effects, such as dyskinesia
- Severe side effects of medications and dementia generally occur within 5 y
- Hallucinations, often of animals or children, are commonly seen in late stages
- In terminal cases, aspiration pneumonia, sepsis, and pulmonary emboli occur
- Physical therapy is often beneficial

42. Progressive Supranuclear Palsy

Etiology/Pathophysiology

- A movement disorder characterized by dystonia, rigidity of axial musculature, and a peculiar disturbance of voluntary eye movements
- An idiopathic degenerative disorder of regions of the midbrain with accumulation of tau protein, neurofibrillary tangles, and senile plaques; pathologically identical to corticobasal ganglionic degeneration
- Mild dementia is generally present
- Presents in mid-to-late life

Differential Dx

- Corticobasal ganglionic degeneration
- Parkinson's disease
- Shy-Drager syndrome

Presentation/Signs & Symptoms

- "Astonished," hyperalert stare
- Impairment of voluntary eye movements requiring the patient to turn entire body to fix gaze
- Dystonic, extended posture of trunk
- Frequent falls with prominent retropulsion
- Dysphagia, dysarthria
- Mild dementia late in course
- Occasional seizures
- Pyramidal signs (e.g., Babinski sign) may be present

Diagnostic Evaluation

- History and physical examination is diagnostic
- No lab test is confirmatory
- MRI may show atrophy of the midbrain region

Treatment/Management

- Treatment is primarily symptomatic
- Dopaminergic agents are minimally helpful
- Tricyclic antidepressants may provide some benefit
- SSRIs for depression

Prognosis/Complications

- Poor prognosis
- Median survival is about 5–8 y
- Death occurs from aspiration pneumonia or secondary to falls

43. Shy-Drager Syndrome

Etiology/Pathophysiology

- A degenerative disorder of the catecholaminergic regions of the basal ganglia, hypothalamus, and autonomic regions of the spinal cord and brainstem that results in severe postural hypotension and rigidity
- Presents with a combination of parkinsonian and cerebellar symptoms with a relative lack of response to dopamine administration
- Loss of intermediolateral horn cells of the spinal cord and pigmented nuclei of the brainstem (sympathetic neurons)
- Etiology is unknown

Differential Dx

- Parkinson's disease
- Vitamin B_{12} deficiency
- Amyloidosis
- Progressive supranuclear palsy
- Olivopontocerebellar atrophy (OPCA)
- Cortico-basal-ganglionic degeneration

Presentation/Signs & Symptoms

- Prominent autonomic symptoms occur early, including profound postural hypotension, diarrhea alternating with constipation, impotence, urinary incontinence or retention, and dry mouth
- Two subtypes: Multiple system atrophy (rigidity and bradykinesia) and OPCA (prominent cerebellar features including ataxia, dysmetria)
- Sleep apnea, stridor, and snoring are prominent

Diagnostic Evaluation

- History and physical examination is diagnostic; must include postural blood pressure measurements
- Autonomic laboratory evaluation including sweat testing and tilt-table testing
- MRI shows changes in the posterolateral putamen

Treatment/Management

- Orthostatic hypotension is treated with fluid and salt administration, reverse Trendelenburg positioning at night, and use of an abdominal binder and Jobst stockings to augment venous return
- Midodrine is an α-agonist used to increase BP
- Fludrocortisone is used to increase salt/water retention
- NSAIDs may be used postprandial hypotension

Prognosis/Complications

- Poor prognosis
- Life expectancy about 5–8 y
- Death generally occurs secondary to aspiration or sepsis

44. Corticobasal Ganglionic Degeneration

Etiology/Pathophysiology

- A degenerative disorder involving the cerebral cortex and basal ganglia that results in impoverished movements and subcortical dementia
- A rare disease that is usually seen by movement disorder specialists usually after treatment for Parkinson's disease failed
- Autopsy shows cortical degeneration with tau protein, neurofibrillatory tangles, Pick bodies, and degeneration of thalamic and basal ganglia neurons
- Pathologically indistinguishable from progressive supranuclear palsy
- Onset begins in the sixth to seventh decades of life

Differential Dx

- Parkinson's disease
- Progressive supranuclear palsy
- Wilson's disease
- Shy-Drager syndrome
- Diffuse Lewy body disease
- Pick's disease
- Alzheimer's disease

Presentation/Signs & Symptoms

- Asymmetrical rigidity
- Postural instability
- Myoclonic tremor
- Dystonic posturing of trunk
- Apraxia
- Cortical sensory dysfunction
- Alien limb (arm moves involuntarily)
- Subcortical dementia
  - Abulia (apathy)
  - Impaired memory
  - Preserved language function

Diagnostic Evaluation

- History and physical examination by a movement disorder specialist is diagnostic; however, the syndrome is difficult to distinguish from other movement disorders
- MRI may show asymmetrical cortical loss and ventriculomegaly

Treatment/Management

- Symptomatic treatment is the only available therapy
- Myoclonus may be treated with clonazepam
- Dementia may be improved with donepezil or memantine
- Some patients respond to dopaminergic agents (e.g., levodopa) to improve movement

Prognosis/Complications

- Progressive disorder with inexorable decline
- 5–10 y life expectancy following diagnosis
- Terminal complications usually include dysphagia, aspiration, and pneumonia

45. Dyskinesia

Etiology/Pathophysiology

- Dyskinesia is defined as abnormal, involuntary movements, usually characterized by continuous motion of the arms, legs, or facial muscles
  - Chorea is a dyskinesia characterized by "dancing" movements of the trunk and extremities; seen in Huntington's and Wilson's disease, Sydenham's chorea, SLE or anti-phospholipid antibody syndrome, pregnancy, OCPs, estrogens, hyper- and hypoparathyroidism
  - Athetosis is a dyskinesia characterized by writhing movements of the extremities; may be seen in cerebral palsy, carbon monoxide poisoning, and kernicterus
  - Ballism is characterized by violent movements of the extremities; often seen following strokes of the subthalamic nuclei
  - Elderly patients often have oral, buccal, or lingual movements
- Dyskinesias are commonly seen in patients with Parkinson's disease who are on chronic dopaminergic medications
- Tardive dyskinesia is a syndrome of oral, facial, and buccal movements that occurs following chronic use of neuroleptic drugs (especially phenothiazines)
- Tourette's syndrome is a dyskinesia characterized by motor and vocal tics with vocalizations and copralalia (yelling out curse words)

Differential Dx

- Dopaminergic effects in Parkinson's patients
- Effect of neuroleptic medication
- Huntington's chorea
- Wilson's disease
- Cerebral palsy
- Tardive dyskinesia
- Tics or habit spasms
- Tourette's syndrome
- Meige's syndrome
- Paroxysmal kinesogenic choreoathetosis

Presentation/Signs & Symptoms

- Chorea: Constant writhing or dancing movements of the trunk, limbs or facial/lingual muscles; disappears during sleep
- Athetosis: Similar to chorea but affects more proximal musculature than chorea
- Ballism: Affects proximal musculature resulting in violent flinging movements
- Oral facial dyskinesias: Eyelid, oral, lingual, and buccal movements, especially in elderly (Meige's syndrome)
- Tics: Stereotyped, repetitive, simple-to-complex motor movements

Diagnostic Evaluation

- Rule out medications, rheumatic fever, SLE, and endocrine disorders
- A workup for Wilson's disease is necessary, including liver function studies, serum ceruloplasmin, and urinary copper
- Genetic testing for Huntington's disease
- Imaging is rarely helpful but will often show basal ganglia abnormalities in Wilson's disease

Treatment/Management

- Remove offending medications if possible
- Treat underlying metabolic or endocrine disorders
- Antidopaminergic agents (e.g., pimozide, haloperidol, risperidone) may improve symptoms in the short term
- Wilson's disease is treated with copper chelators and zinc administration

Prognosis/Complications

- Symptoms of Tourette's syndrome may disappear with time
- Dyskinesias may persist despite removal of the offending medication
- Wilson's disease may improve dramatically after chelation therapy, although cirrhosis and dyskinesias may persist

46. Dystonia

Etiology/Pathophysiology

- An abnormal movement with a fixed, usually twisted, posture of the limbs or axial musculature
- Most commonly idiopathic or posttraumatic
- Often induced by neuroleptic medications (e.g., phenothiazines) or drugs with strong antidopaminergic activity (e.g., compazine)
- May be of autosomal dominant (DTY-1 gene) or recessive inheritance (torsion dystonia)
- Psychogenic factors may play a role

Differential Dx

- Wilson's disease
- Torticollis (wry neck)
- Progressive supranuclear palsy
- Torsion dystonia
- Cerebral palsy
- Advanced Parkinson's disease
- Childhood Huntington's disease
- Excessive dopaminergic activity
- Psychogenic dystonia

Presentation/Signs & Symptoms

- Trunk or limbs are twisted into a firm, usually hyperextended posture
- Fixed smile, lingual posturing
- Blepharospasm may be present with various types of dystonia or may occur alone: Forced eye closures or frequent blinking
- Torticollis: Forced deviation of the head to one side due to over contraction of the contralateral sternomastoid; may be fixed or spasmodic

Diagnostic Evaluation

- History and physical examination is generally diagnostic
- MRI of brain to exclude basal ganglia abnormalities
- Rule out Wilson's disease with serum ceruloplasmin and urinary copper level

Treatment/Management

- Discontinue offending medications if possible
- If dystonia is induced by drugs, administration of diphenhydramine (Benadryl) IM or IV will relieve symptoms
- Botox injections may be effective for blepharospasm, torticollis, and other forms of dystonia, especially if painful
- Dopamine agonists (e.g., levodopa) or anticholinergics (e.g., trihexyphenidyl, benztropine) are sometimes effective
- For extreme dystonia, oral or intrathecal lioresal may be used
- Thalamotomy or pallidotomy are sometimes used in extreme cases
- Deep brain stimulation may be used

Prognosis/Complications

- Generalized symptoms or younger age of onset generally results in a worse prognosis

47. Essential Tremor

Etiology/Pathophysiology

- A common tremor that is more pronounced when trying to maintain a posture
- Characterized by 8–12 per min rhythmic movements of the hands, palate, or head
- May have autosomal dominant inheritance
- Age of onset variable but generally seen in late life
- No known underlying pathology
- Disappears during sleep
- Worsened with caffeine and anxiety
- Relieved by alcohol ingestion

Differential Dx

- Parkinson's disease
- Anxiety
- Thyrotoxicosis
- Wilson's disease
- Medications (e.g., β-agonists, lithium, amiodarone, valproic acid)
- Action myoclonus

Presentation/Signs & Symptoms

- Seen primarily when trying to maintain a posture or action
- Affects handwriting and feeding
- Limbs, head (e.g., head nodding, shaking "no"), and voice are commonly involved
- Can be differentiated from Parkinson's disease in that the tremor normally does not occur substantially at rest and the head and voice are not similarly affected in Parkinson's disease

Diagnostic Evaluation

- History and physical examination is generally diagnostic
- Check serum ceruloplasmin and urinary copper levels to rule out Wilson's disease, especially in younger patients
- Thyroid function studies to exclude thyrotoxicosis

Treatment/Management

- Mild cases do not require treatment
- Medical therapy can be used as needed (e.g., during social events)
- Primidone and propranolol are the most commonly used agents to decrease the tremor
- Other agents may include topiramate, mirtazapine, and methazolamine
- Surgical therapy may be considered in severe cases but is rarely necessary, including thalamotomy or thalamic deep brain stimulation

Prognosis/Complications

- Usually not disabling but may be socially embarrassing
- May worsen with time but patients should be assured that they do not have a life-threatening disorder
- Patients should be discouraged from using alcohol, even though they may experience benefit

48. Huntington's Disease

Etiology/Pathophysiology

- An inherited disorder associated with abnormal involuntary movements and dementia
- Caused by an autosomal dominant mutation in chromosome 4 that results in increased CAG repeats (spontaneous mutations also occur)
- Results in a loss of GABA neurons in the caudate and putamen
- Movement disorder that affects the basal ganglia and frontal lobes
- Typical age of onset is 35–40 y old, but may be earlier in severe cases—age of onset can be predicted by the number of CAG repeats in chromosome 4 (the more repeats, the earlier the onset of symptoms)

Differential Dx

- Sydenham's chorea
- Dopaminergic-induced chorea
- Medication-induced dystonia or dyskinesia
- Cerebral palsy with dystonic movements
- Parkinson's disease
- Wilson's disease
- Various causes of dementia (e.g., Alzheimer's disease, Pick's disease, infectious and metabolic causes)

Presentation/Signs & Symptoms

- Psychiatric symptoms often precede chorea
- Erratic behavior, loss of forbearance, self-control, temper outbursts
- Poor judgment, loss of acquired skills, slowness in completing tasks
- Clumsiness, stumbling gait
- Involuntary movements, chorea of arms and legs
- Patient may try to obscure movements by crossing legs or placing hand on mouth
- Severe depression and suicide common
- Voice and speech dystonic with inability to control amplitude or volume
- Childhood onset may be dystonic or rigid (rare)

Diagnostic Evaluation

- History and physical examination with careful family history is imperative
- Lab and CSF studies are normal
- CT or MRI may show cerebral and caudate atrophy
- EEG shows diffuse changes
- Diagnosis can be made on the basis of genetic testing; however, careful consideration must be given to screening unaffected family members since there is no way to alter the course of the disease

Treatment/Management

- No known cure and no treatment is available to slow the progress
- Initial efforts can be made to control the choreic movements with neuroleptics, haloperidol, or reserpine
- Coenzyme Q_{10} may be tried
- Valproic acid may improve emotional symptoms
- Psychotherapy and antidepressants for depression

Prognosis/Complications

- Progressive dementia and chorea occurs
- Average life expectancy 15–20 y from diagnosis
- Suicide occurs in up to 20% of cases
- Terminally, patients may become rigid
- Death may occur due to pneumonia as patients are unable to clear secretions
- Eventually, voluntary movements become very difficult and the personality changes lead to the need for institutionalization

49. Wilson's Disease

Etiology/Pathophysiology

- Also known as hepatolenticular degeneration
- An inherited disorder of copper metabolism resulting in copper overload and deposition in multiple tissues
- The disorder principally consists of hepatic cirrhosis and degeneration of the basal ganglia
- Autosomal recessive inheritance
- Pathophysiology involves impaired binding of copper to ceruloplasmin, the body's copper binding protein
- Free copper accumulates in organs including brain, cornea, liver, and kidneys
- Disease often begins in teenage years with psychiatric, hepatic, and neurologic presentations

Differential Dx

- Parkinson's disease
- Drug-induced dystonias
- Huntington's disease
- Essential tremor

Presentation/Signs & Symptoms

- Dystonic facial posture with fixed grimace or smile
- Postural tremor
- Ataxia
- Personality changes
- Asterixis or "wing-beating" tremor
- Hepatitis, cirrhosis, and jaundice
- Kayser-Fleischer rings in the cornea due to copper deposits; may only be seen with slit-lamp examination (only present if neurologic signs exist)
- Dysphagia and dysarthria
- Occasional pyramidal signs (e.g., spasticity, Babinski sign)
- Mild cognitive disturbances

Diagnostic Evaluation

- History and physical examination
  - Presence of Kayser-Fleischer rings on slit-lamp examination is diagnostic
- MRI or CT shows increased signal in the basal ganglia or dentate nuclei; occasional cystic changes in the basal ganglia are seen
- Reduced serum copper and ceruloplasmin levels
- Increased urinary copper
- Abnormal liver function enzymes

Treatment/Management

- Restriction of dietary copper ingestion (e.g., liver, mushrooms, chocolate, shellfish)
- Copper chelation therapy (penicillamine) should be started as soon as diagnosed
- Zinc is also used, which blocks the intestinal absorption of copper

Prognosis/Complications

- Treatment with chelation therapy should be life-long
- Improvement is expected in most cases
- Many patients are cured, but others have permanent hepatic or cerebral dysfunction

Demyelinating Disorders

JON BRILLMAN, MD, FRCPI
THOMAS F. SCOTT, MD

Section 6

50. Multiple Sclerosis

Etiology/Pathophysiology

- Relatively common acquired demyelinating disease of young adults that can follow a relapsing/remitting course with variable degrees of disability
- Presumed to be an autoimmune process; some evidence suggests that the disease is contracted in early life when a viral antigen stimulates the immune system, resulting in complex B and T cell dysregulation
- Affects CNS and optic nerves
- Destruction of myelin sheaths results in demyelination and inflammation of CNS white matter; multiple plaques of demyelination of different ages and in different locations are seen ("separated by both time and space")
- Unknown etiology; probably an autoimmune process that occurs in genetically susceptible persons
    - Familial incidence of about 15% suggesting an infectious etiology
    - There are certain histocompatibility antigens in patients with multiple sclerosis suggesting a genetic predisposition
- Peak onset ages 20–40; rarely occurs after 50
- Increasing incidence with increasing latitude: <1/100,000 at the equator; up to 80/100,000 in northern U.S. and Canada
- Females are affected slightly more commonly than males
- 50% of patients with optic neuritis will go on to develop multiple sclerosis

Differential Dx

- Acute disseminated encephalomyelitis
- Other demyelinating syndromes (e.g., central pontine myelinolysis, Devic's disease, Baló's disease)
- Autoimmune disorders (e.g., SLE, vasculitis, antiphospholipid antibody syndrome, sarcoidosis)
- Neoplastic and paraneoplastic syndromes (especially lymphoma)
- Gliomatosis cerebri
- Adrenoleukodystrophy
- Metachromatic leukodystrophy
- HIV encephalopathy
- Vitamin B_{12} deficiency

Presentation/Signs & Symptoms

- Optic (retrobulbar) neuritis: Visual loss
- Myelitis (Lhermitte sign is a sensation of electricity down the back upon passive flexion of the neck)
- Brainstem and cerebellar dysfunction: Diplopia, ataxia, dysarthria, dysmetria
- Weakness: Monoparesis, hemiparesis, or paraparesis
- Sensory symptoms may include sensory level in spinal cord disease
- Bladder/bowel dysfunction
- Psychiatric features include depression, cognitive complaints
- Marcus-Gunn pupil
- Ophthalmoplegia
- Upper motor neuron signs (e.g., Babinski, hyperreflexia)

Diagnostic Evaluation

- History, exam, and ancillary tests determine the likelihood of disease as "clinically definite," "lab-supported definite," "clinically probable," or "lab-supported probable"
- MRI with T2 weighting and FLAIR is the most sensitive test; shows multiple white matter abnormalities in periventricular location
    - For patients with classic demyelinating lesions on MRI, minimal additional workup needed
    - Multifocal demyelinating lesions separated in "space and time" are present
    - If lesions not seen, the diagnosis should be reconsidered
    - In patients with optic neuritis, if the MRI reveals typical lesions of MS, the full disease will likely develop
- CSF reveals oligoclonal bands and increased IgG; mild lymphocytic pleocytosis in acute attacks; protein may be mildly elevated
- Slowed evoked potentials (visual, auditory, and sensory)

Treatment/Management

- There is no cure for MS, but existing therapies often give good results
- Steroids are indicated for acute attacks (high-dose IV steroids for moderate-to-severe attacks, low-dose oral steroids for mild attacks)
- Immunomodulators (e.g., interferons, glatiramer acetate) for prophylaxis of relapsing events
- Consider IVIG or plasmapheresis for unusually severe attacks
- Consider immunosuppressive agents and chemotherapy for unusually severe progressive cases
- Supportive care includes physical therapy, prostheses/orthotics, amantadine to reduce fatigue, antispasmodics (e.g., baclofen), antidepressants, bladder dysfunction agents (e.g., oxybutynin), and analgesia
- Natalizumab IV has recently been approved for relapsing-remitting disease

Prognosis/Complications

- Course marked by exacerbations and remissions: Relapsing remitting (episodes of acute worsening and recovery), secondary progressive (gradual deterioration with superimposed relapses), primary progressive (gradual deterioration from onset), progressive relapsing (gradual deterioration from onset with additional relapses)
- Predictive factors are weak but identifiable (worse prognosis in male gender, later onset, progressive form from onset, motor symptoms from onset, poor recovery from first attack)
- MRI is weakly predictive (many lesions suggest worse prognosis)
- Patients who do well in the first 5 y tend to do well for the next 5–10 y or longer; those who do well for the first 10 y have a 90% chance of doing well for another 10 y

51. Optic Neuritis

Etiology/Pathophysiology

- An inflammatory demyelination of optic nerve resulting in varying degrees of central vision loss
- May be idiopathic
- Often presents as a manifestation of multiple sclerosis
- Infrequently seen as a manifestation of connective tissue disease, autoimmune diseases, or postviral inflammation
- 50% of patients with optic or retrobulbar neuritis will develop multiple sclerosis

Differential Dx

- Multiple sclerosis
- Acute demyelinating encephalomyelitis
- Devic's disease (simultaneous bilateral optic neuritis, myelitis)
- Autoimmune diseases (e.g., SLE, sarcoidosis)
- Vasculitis
- Paraneoplastic or neoplastic disease
- Anterior ischemic optic neuropathy
- Central retinal artery occlusion
- Amaurosis fugax
- Leber's optic atrophy
- Transient obscurations due to papilledema

Presentation/Signs & Symptoms

- Often initially presents with eye pain that occurs with or without movement
- Central visual field loss
  - May be mild to severe
  - Red desaturation (poor color vision)
- Afferent pupillary defect (Marcus-Gunn pupil)
- Progresses over minutes to weeks
- Upper motor neuron signs, brainstem dysfunction, or other abnormalities on neurologic exam may suggest a second demyelinating lesion or multiple sclerosis

Diagnostic Evaluation

- Detailed history and review of systems to identify previous neurologic events or symptoms of systemic disease
- Cerebral MRI with T2 weighting and FLAIR to evaluate optic nerves and brain
- CSF reveals oligoclonal bands and increased IgG; mild lymphocytic pleocytosis in acute attacks; protein may be mildly elevated
- Slowed visual evoked potentials
- Screening for connective tissue disease may include ESR, ANA, SS-A antibodies, anticardiolipin antibodies, angiotensin converting enzyme, C-ANCA antibodies, and paraneoplastic antibodies
- For patients with classic demyelinating lesions on MRI scan, minimal additional workup is needed
- Ophthalmologic evaluation, including central visual fields

Treatment/Management

- Steroids are controversial but are generally administered (high doses for moderate-to-severe disease, varying doses for milder disease)
  - It is unclear whether steroids prevent subsequent development of multiple sclerosis
- Consider IVIG or plasmapheresis for severe, steroid refractory, bilateral disease
- Consider immunosuppressives for severe recurrent disease
- Immunomodulators for cases associated with MS

Prognosis/Complications

- Nearly 90% of patients have full recovery of vision or at least 20/30 visual acuity
- If cerebral MRI suggests MS at the onset of optic neuritis, 50–90% will develop multiple sclerosis within 5–10 y
- If cerebral MRI is negative at onset of optic neuritis, 10% will develop multiple sclerosis within 5 y and 20% within 10 y

52. Acute Disseminated Encephalomyelitis

Etiology/Pathophysiology

- An idiopathic inflammatory disorder generally classified as a demyelinating disease
- Presumably of autoimmune origin; likely due to a hypersensitivity reaction
- Usually preceded by a viral illness or *Mycoplasma* infection 2–6 weeks
- A rare disorder, perhaps 1 per 100,000 prevalence in the U.S.
- More common in children than adults
- Associated with perivascular lymphocytic cuffs, demyelination, and usually large focal areas of cerebral edema with breakdown of the blood-brain barrier
- Occurs as a monophasic disease (a single event); Multiple sclerosis should be considered as the diagnosis if recurrent demyelinating events occur
- Demyelination may involve the spinal cord
- The most severe form is acute necrotizing hemorrhagic encephalomyelitis

Differential Dx

- Multiple sclerosis
- Other demyelinating syndromes (e.g., central pontine myelinolysis, Baló's disease)
- Connective tissue disease and autoimmune disorders (e.g., sarcoidosis, Wegener's granulomatous, and other forms of vasculitis)
- Gliomatosis cerebri
- Cerebral abscess
- Metastatic cerebral lesions
- Cerebral lymphoma

Presentation/Signs & Symptoms

- Generally presents with ataxia, encephalopathy, focal and generalized weakness, myelopathy (e.g., paraplegia), brainstem dysfunction (e.g., diplopia, dysarthria), sensory symptoms, bowel and bladder dysfunction, optic neuritis (loss of vision), ophthalmoplegia, and upper motor neuron signs (e.g., Babinski sign, hyperreflexia)
- Seizures occur in about 20% of cases
- Fever (in the absence of infection) occurs in about 20% of cases

Diagnostic Evaluation

- Head and spinal MRI with T2 weighting and FLAIR generally reveals several large, rounded, edematous lesions with variable degrees and patterns of contrast enhancement
- CSF analysis reveals oligoclonal bands, IgG index, pleocytosis (increased cells), and mildly elevated protein
- Consider screening for connective tissue diseases: ESR, ANA, c-ANCA antibodies, angiotensin converting enzyme
- Consider chest X-ray or CT to rule out sarcoidosis and cancer
- Consider brain biopsy if the diagnosis is in question

Treatment/Management

- High-dose IV steroids for 3–5 d
- Plasmapheresis is indicated for patients who fail steroids
- Consider cyclophosphamide or other immunosuppressive agents if all else fails

Prognosis/Complications

- Patients tend to recover fully; however, those with spinal cord involvement are especially prone to residual weakness
- Rarely, severe hemorrhagic forms of the disease are fatal
- Rarely considered to be recurrent; however, occasionally recurrences have been seen
    - Recurrent demyelinating events should prompt an evaluation for multiple sclerosis
- In all cases, it is uncertain whether or not a patient will go on to develop MS (i.e., suffer recurrent attacks of demyelination); in typical cases of acute disseminated encephalomyelitis, it appears unlikely that patients will go on to develop MS

53. Transverse Myelitis

Etiology/Pathophysiology

- An idiopathic inflammatory disorder of the spinal cord normally occurring in the thoracic region and resulting in paraparesis, paraplegia, and sensory levels
- May be primary or secondary to a more specific inflammatory disorder (e.g., MS, connective tissue diseases)
- Usually a monophasic disease (single event)
- Idiopathic transverse myelitis is felt to be due to an autoimmune delayed type IV hypersensitivity reaction following a viral or bacterial infection
- Perivenular lymphocytic cuffing is seen on pathology, essentially indistinguishable from MS at the microscopic level
- Incidence not certain, probably in the range of 1 case per 100,000

Differential Dx

- Other demyelinating diseases (e.g., MS)
- Devic's disease (simultaneous bilateral optic neuritis and myelitis)
- Spinal cord infarct
- Mass lesions
- Vitamin B_{12} deficiency
- Sarcoidosis
- SLE
- Sjögren's syndrome
- Vasculitis
- Antiphospholipid antibody syndrome
- Severe disk herniation or other compressive lesions
- Radiation myelitis

Presentation/Signs & Symptoms

- Classically follows a subacute course, evolving over several days
- Severe spinal cord dysfunction referable to a cervical or thoracic level with bilateral symptoms (complete transverse myelitis), or hemicord syndromes (e.g., Brown-Séquard syndrome, acute partial transverse myelitis)
- Sensory, complete transverse, or hemisensory level
- Less commonly presents as ascending numbness with ill-defined sensory level
- Bladder and bowel dysfunction (urinary retention, urgency, and frequency)
- Hyperreflexia is usually present
- Babinski sign
- Interscapular pain may occur

Diagnostic Evaluation

- MRI of the spinal cord with and without contrast
  - Follow-up spinal MRI for patients with poor recovery or suspicious MRI lesions (rule out spinal cord tumors)
- MRI of the brain to rule out MS with asymptomatic cerebral lesions
  - Follow-up cerebral MRI in patients with idiopathic myelitis to monitor for possible development of MS
- CSF analysis may reveal oligoclonal bands and elevated IgG
- Autoimmunity workup includes ANA, anticardiolipin antibodies, SS-A antibodies, ESR, c-ANCA and p-ANCA antibodies, and vitamin B_{12} level

Treatment/Management

- Observation is sufficient for patients with minimal dysfunction
- High-dose corticosteroids for patients with moderate-to-severe dysfunction
- Specific therapy as indicated for any specific diagnosis found during workup

Prognosis/Complications

- Most cases of transverse myelitis, either complete or partial, have excellent recoveries
- Patients with severe complete idiopathic transverse myelitis have less than 5% chance of developing MS
- Patients with idiopathic acute partial transverse myelitis have 10–20% chance of developing MS; should be monitored (much higher risk if MRI of cerebrum consistent with MS at presentation)
- Patients with idiopathic myelitis have a slight chance (perhaps 1%) of developing a connective tissue disease, Devic's, or other autoimmune illness, and should be followed accordingly with routine checkups
- 5–10% of patients may relapse with a similar or more severe bout of myelitis, also idiopathic (idiopathic relapsing transverse myelitis)

54. Progressive Multifocal Leukoencephalopathy

Etiology/Pathophysiology

- A viral demyelinating disorder seen exclusively in immunosuppressed patients (e.g., transplant recipients, AIDS patients, leukemia/lymphoma)
- Caused by reactivation of latent JC virus in immunosuppressed or immunocompromised patients
    - 90% of all humans are infected with JC virus at a young age
- See also *AIDS and the Nervous System*

Differential Dx

- CNS lymphoma
- Acute disseminated encephalomyelitis
- CNS HIV infection
- Microvascular ischemic cerebral disease (e.g., Binswanger's disease)
- Gliomatosis cerebri
- Adrenoleukodystrophy
- Metachromatic leukodystrophy

Presentation/Signs & Symptoms

- Rapidly progressive clinical course
- Visual loss
- Dysarthria
- Confusion
- Aphasia
- Dementia
- Ataxia
- Hemiparesis
- Seizures occur uncommonly, usually late in the course of disease

Diagnostic Evaluation

- MRI with T2 weighting and FLAIR reveals multifocal areas of nonenhancing hyperintensities; may involve cerebral hemispheres, brainstem, cerebellum, and/or spinal cord
- JC virus DNA can be detected by PCR in the CSF
- CSF is otherwise unremarkable
- Brain biopsy reveals demyelination with viral particles within oligodendrocyte nuclei demonstrated by electron microscopy; giant astrocytes are frequently seen

Treatment/Management

- No cure is available
- May respond to interferons or cytosine arabinoside

Prognosis/Complications

- Ultimately leads to coma and death within 1 y in 90% of cases

55. Central Pontine Myelinolysis

Etiology/Pathophysiology

- A demyelinating disorder primarily of the pons that occurs in patients with immunocompromise, nutritional deficiencies, or electrolyte imbalances
  - Seen in alcoholics and patients with systemic cancer
  - Seen with vitamin deficiencies, especially thiamine
  - Also occurs as a result of overly aggressive correction of hyponatremia
- Pathophysiology is felt to be related to osmotic changes that result in demyelination
- Diamond-shaped lesions in the pons are most commonly seen but lesions may be extrapontine
- Destruction of the myelin sheaths occur, with preservation of axons
- Sporadic occurrence

Differential Dx

- Acute disseminated encephalomyelitis
- MS, other demyelinating syndromes (Devic's, Baló's disease)
- Autoimmune disorders (SLE, vasculitis, antiphospholipid antibody syndrome, sarcoidosis)
- Neoplastic, paraneoplastic syndromes (especially lymphoma)
- Gliomatosis cerebri
- Adrenoleukodystrophy
- Metachromatic leukodystrophy
- HIV encephalopathy
- Vitamin B_{12} deficiency
- Basilar artery occlusion

Presentation/Signs & Symptoms

- Subacute onset of quadriparesis or quadriplegia
- Dysarthria
- Dysphagia
- Bilateral facial weakness
- Nystagmus
- Bilateral Babinski signs
- "Locked-in" state (patient is quadriplegic and awake with an inability to move eyes horizontally)

Diagnostic Evaluation

- MRI scan with T2 weighting and FLAIR shows a large quadrangular lesion in mid-pons; extrapontine lesions may be seen
- Slow auditory evoked potentials
- CSF is unremarkable

Treatment/Management

- Correction of hyponatremia should be slow at rate of 10 mEq per liter per day
- Vitamin replacement, especially vitamins B_1 and B_{12}
- Supportive care, including intubation if necessary

Prognosis/Complications

- Prognosis is poor, but with excellent care patients may survive with minimal disability

Infections of the Central Nervous System

JON BRILLMAN, MD, FRCPI

56. Bacterial Meningitis

Etiology/Pathophysiology

- Infection typically occurs via the bloodstream from mucosal reservoirs (e.g., nasopharynx, respiratory tract, GI tract, genital tract), may also occur by contiguous spread (e.g., otitis media, skull fracture)
- The most commonly involved bacteria are *Streptococcus pneumoniae*, *Neisseria meningitidis*, and *Haemophilus influenzae*
- Adults: *S. pneumoniae*, *N. meningitidis*, *Listeria monocytogenes*
  - *S. pneumoniae*: Gram-positive diplococcus; spreads from nasopharynx to bloodstream to meninges in adults, especially those with mild immunosuppression (e.g., diabetes, alcoholism, HIV infection, chronic sinusitis, middle ear infections, old age)
  - *N. meningitidis*: Gram-negative diplococcus; colonized in nasopharynx, can rapidly spread to bloodstream in susceptible individuals; may cause epidemic meningitis, or may be spontaneous or isolated
  - *Listeria monocytogenes*: Weakly gram-positive; often seen in immunocompromised individuals, but may be sporadic
- Children: *H. influenzae* was common, now rare due to vaccination
- Neonates: *E. coli*
- Neonates and pregnant females: Group B streptococcus

Differential Dx

- Viral meningitis
- Fungal meningitis
- Tuberculous meningitis
- Herpes simplex encephalitis
- Viral infections that present with myalgias
- Brain abscess
- Subdural empyema
- Sepsis
- Meningeal carcinomatosis

Presentation/Signs & Symptoms

- Classic triad of fever, headache, and meningismus (stiff neck)
- Cerebral dysfunction, beginning with confusion and possibly progressing to stupor and coma
- Delirium
- Seizures
- Cranial nerve dysfunction (e.g., diplopia)
- In cases of *N. meningitidis*, sepsis and circulatory collapse may occur catastrophically before meningeal infection becomes apparent
- Petechiae and purpura may occur, particularly in *N. meningitidis* meningitis

Diagnostic Evaluation

- Initial studies include CBC, blood cultures, and chest X-ray
- CT scan should initially be used to rule out brain edema with increased intracranial pressure or mass lesion; however, imaging should not delay a lumbar puncture if meningitis is strongly suspected
- Lumbar puncture with CSF analysis is the key to diagnosis
  - Manifested by a reactive pleocytosis (increased cells)
  - WBCs are markedly elevated (although may be few early)
  - >90% PMNs are usually present; however, *Listeria* shows fewer numbers of cells and high lymphocyte count
  - Protein is usually >100 mg/dL
  - CSF glucose is less than 50% of blood glucose
  - Gram stain must be evaluated emergently
  - Obtain cultures with sensitivities
  - PCR detection of bacterial DNA may be helpful
- MRI with contrast may reveal brain edema, abnormal meningeal enhancement; sinuses usually visualized

Treatment/Management

- Rapid administration of empiric IV antimicrobials that achieve high levels within the CSF is essential
  - Vancomycin plus either ceftriaxone, cefotaxime, or meropenum is a treatment of choice
- Narrow the antibiotics once organism is identified
  - *S. pneumoniae*: Ceftriaxone, cefotaxime, or penicillin for 2 wk
  - *N. meningitidis*: Penicillin, ampicillin, or ceftriaxone for 7–10 d
  - *Listeria*: Ampicillin plus gentamicin for 14–21 d
  - *H. influenzae*: Ceftriaxone or chloramphenicol for 7–10 d
  - Group B streptococcus: Penicillin, ampicillin, or vancomycin for 14–21 d
- Corticosteroid administration is optional if significant brain edema is present
- Rifampin prophylaxis in any individual exposed to *N. meningitidis* infection

Prognosis/Complications

- Mortality is 15–25% in adults, 5–15% in children
- Complications are extremely common and include stroke, cerebral edema, hydrocephalus, sepsis and septic shock, DIC, and ARDS
- Vaccines are available for *H. influenzae*, *S. pneumoniae*, and *N. meningitidis*
- *N. meningitidis* bacteremia precedes meningeal involvement and may be very severe, potentially resulting in death from circulatory collapse; this should be recognized by purpura or petechiae on skin and associated hypotension; loss of limbs are a potential sequelae secondary to gangrene
- Cranial nerve dysfunction, including deafness, may occur, especially in children
- Epilepsy occurs in less than 10% of cases

57. Viral & Aseptic Meningitis

Etiology/Pathophysiology

- Meningitis is an inflammation of the leptomeninges (pia and arachnoid) secondary to infectious or chemical agents
- Viral meningitis is a benign condition associated with upper respiratory infections
    - Most cases are associated with herpes simplex virus-2, enterovirus, arbovirus, mumps, varicella, and Epstein-Barr viruses
    - Usually lasts about a week
- Aseptic meningitis is a benign inflammation of the leptomeninges which may be caused by an infectious agent
    - Has been associated with medications (e.g., anti-inflammatory drugs, IVIG), Behçet's syndrome, Mollaret's disease, and sarcoidosis

Differential Dx

- Bacterial meningitis
- Migraine
- Viral infections with associated myalgias
- Meningeal carcinomatosis
- Fungal or tuberculous meningitis
- Encephalitis
- Brain abscess
- Subdural empyema

Presentation/Signs & Symptoms

- The presentation differs from bacterial meningitis in that it is less severe and there is no associated encephalopathy
- Headache
- Meningismus
- Fever (frequently low grade)
- Nausea/vomiting
- Photophobia
- Malaise
- Myalgias

Diagnostic Evaluation

- Initial studies include CBC, chest X-ray, and blood cultures
- CT initially to rule out brain edema in increased intracranial pressure or mass lesion; however, imaging should not delay a lumbar puncture if meningitis is strongly suspected
- Lumbar puncture with CSF analysis is the key to diagnosis
    - Manifested by a reactive pleocytosis (increased cells); however, the number and types of cells differ from bacterial meningitis
    - WBCs are only mildly elevated
    - PMNs may be elevated early (up to 85%), but then lymphocytes become the predominant cell type
    - Protein is normal or mildly elevated (usually <100 mg/dL)
    - CSF glucose is normal
    - Gram stain and bacterial cultures are negative PCR may identify specific viral DNA
- Imaging is generally normal

Treatment/Management

- Treatment is primarily supportive
    - Antipyretic and analgesic medications
    - Rehydration is often necessary
- Removal of offending agent in the case of medication-induced meningitis

Prognosis/Complications

- Complete recovery is expected
- Recurrent meningitis occurs in about 10% of cases, especially in cases of repeated NSAID use and herpes simplex virus-2
- Repeat lumbar puncture is optional

58. Herpes Simplex Encephalitis

Etiology/Pathophysiology

- Encephalitis is an inflammation of the brain parenchyma
- Viral infections are the most common etiology
- HSV-1 is the most common cause of acute viral encephalitis and is associated with a high mortality rate if untreated
- Primary HSV-1 infection occurs in the oropharynx and becomes latent in the trigeminal ganglia
- Reactivation of the virus at a later time results in brain infection via retrograde transmission of the virus to the temporal lobes and orbitofrontal areas
- The cause of the reactivation is largely unknown but may occasionally be related to immunosuppression
- Rarely, cases may be caused by primary infection

Differential Dx

- Arbovirus encephalitis
- Rabies encephalitis
- Aseptic meningitis
- Meningeal carcinomatosis
- Bacterial meningitis
- Fungal and tubercular meningoencephalitis

Presentation/Signs & Symptoms

- Fever (up to 104°F [40.0°C])
- Headache
- Altered consciousness (e.g., confusion, stupor, coma) possible secondary to increased intracranial pressure
- Seizures (complex partial and generalized) occur frequently
- Aphasia if the dominant hemisphere is involved
- Personality changes (e.g., hypersexuality, hallucinations)
- Hemiparesis
- Meningismus may be present

Diagnostic Evaluation

- Initial laboratory examination: CBC, blood cultures, and chest X-ray
- Head CT or MRI will demonstrate edema and a necrotic mass in the temporal lobe or orbitofrontal gyri
- Lumbar puncture with CSF reveals pleocytosis (increased cells)
    - Unlike other viral meningitides where PMNs may predominate early, lymphocytes are the predominant cell type (20–500 cells/mm^3)
    - RBCs are prominent due to necrosis of brain tissue
    - Protein is elevated
    - Glucose is usually normal
    - PCR for HSV-1 DNA is positive from weeks 1–4 and has very high sensitivity and specificity
    - HSV antibody is detected in 90% of cases
- Brain biopsy is no longer required for diagnosis

Treatment/Management

- Immediate treatment with IV acylovir is essential as soon as the diagnosis is suspected to reduce morbidity and mortality
    - Treatment is continued for 3 wk
- Corticosteroids may be used to control excessive brain edema
- Supportive care may include mechanical ventilation, electrolyte management, and anticonvulsant therapy (phenytoin is commonly used)

Prognosis/Complications

- 70% mortality rate if untreated
- 60% cure rate is expected if acyclovir is started early
- 20% mortality even with treatment
- 20% of patients have residual symptoms including complex partial seizures, memory impairment, or disinhibition (e.g., inappropriate sexual behavior)

59. Arbovirus Encephalitis

Etiology/Pathophysiology

- Encephalitis is an inflammation of the brain parenchyma
- Arboviruses are transmitted by arthropods, usually mosquitoes
  - The virus is introduced into the host by a mosquito bite with subsequent viremia
  - Animals are often reservoirs, including birds and horses
  - There is often a geographic prevalence
- There is usually a seasonal incidence; most common in late summer and early fall
- Infection is blood borne to brain capillaries and then spreads to neurons in the spinal cord and neurons in the gray matter
- The leptomeninges are commonly inflamed
- Common types include California or La Crosse, St. Louis, Japanese B, Eastern Equine, Western Equine, and, more recently, West Nile virus
- All types of arbovirus encephalitis may be epidemic

Differential Dx

- Other etiologies of encephalitis (e.g., HSV-1, poliomyelitis)
- Aseptic or viral meningitis
- Guillain-Barré syndrome
- Bacterial meningitis
- Fungal or tubercular meningitis
- Rabies

Presentation/Signs & Symptoms

- A prodrome of headache, fever, and vomiting occurs
- Altered level of consciousness (confusion, stupor, coma)
- Seizures (focal and generalized) are usually present
- West Nile virus may additionally cause an asymmetrical quadraparesis and respiratory failure with loss of deep tendon reflexes (similar to poliomyelitis)

Diagnostic Evaluation

- Head MRI with T2 weighting may reveal bright signals in the basal ganglia or thalamus
- Lumbar puncture with CSF analysis reveals typical findings of viral infections
  - Pleocytosis (increased cells) 20–500 cells/mm^3
  - PMNs may be prominent early but then lymphocytes become the predominate cell type
  - Protein is mildly elevated or normal; glucose is normal
  - Viral-specific IgM antibody has high sensitivity/specificity
  - Virus is rarely cultured from the CSF
- Definitive diagnosis is made by acute and convalescent serologies in the blood
- Brain biopsy may be necessary to confirm viral etiology
  - Pathology reveals intranuclear inclusion bodies and perivascular lymphocytes
- Electrodiagnostic studies confirm lower motor neuron lesions in West Nile virus infections

Treatment/Management

- Treatment is primarily supportive, including IV fluids, electrolyte management, control of seizures, and possible mechanical ventilation
- Antiviral drugs are of no benefit

Prognosis/Complications

- Mortality is high, especially in cases of Eastern Equine encephalitis
- Residual neurologic deficits may occur in up to 40% of cases
- Seizures may persist

60. Brain Abscess

Etiology/Pathophysiology

- Brain abscesses rare, associated with infections of other parts of the body
  - About half of cases arise from sinus, middle ear, and mastoid infections; these spread to the brain via bone (osteomyelitis) or venous tracts
  - The remainder of cases are secondary to penetrating cranial trauma, periodontal or pulmonary infections, infective endocarditis, and GI tract infections; these metastatic abscesses arise from hematogenous spread
- Ear and sinus infections spread to temporal lobe or cerebellum, whereas hematogenous infections spread to the deep brain structures or arterial territories
- The most common organisms in brain abscesses include microaerophilic or anaerobic streptococci mixed with other organisms (e.g., *Bacteroides*, *E. coli*, *Proteus*)
  - Staphylococcal infections may result from penetrating injuries to the skull
- Increased risk in immunocompromised patients (e.g., *Toxoplasma*)
- 20% of cases are cryptogenic
- Abscesses are common in children with congenital heart disease
- According to CT scans, abscesses have an early cerebritis phase followed by an encapsulated phase, which may take 4–6 wk to develop

Differential Dx

- Subdural empyema
- Intracranial mass lesion (e.g., neoplasm)
- Meningitis
- Herpes simplex encephalitis
- Cerebral hematoma

Presentation/Signs & Symptoms

- Headache
- Lethargy
- Fever/chills
- Seizures
- Focal neurological deficits (e.g., arm/leg weakness)
- Signs of increased intracranial pressure (e.g., hiccups, diplopia, papilledema, stupor, coma)

Diagnostic Evaluation

- History and physical exam, including detailed neurologic examination
- Laboratory studies include CBC with differential (reveals leukocytosis), blood cultures, and C-reactive protein (often elevated)
- Chest X-ray, chest CT, and sinus X-rays are often indicated
- Head CT and MRI with contrast may reveal a ring-enhancing lesion with extensive edema
  - Early findings include hypodensity on CT, hypointensity on T1-weighted MRI, and hyperintensity on T2-weighted MRI
  - The later encapsulated phase shows ring enhancement and edema
- CT- or MRI-guided aspiration and biopsy may yield a diagnosis in difficult cases

Treatment/Management

- Administer appropriate IV antibiotics or antifungals for 4–6 wk
  - Most abscesses are mixed flora and are usually microaerophilic: Use vancomycin, third-generation cephalosporins, and metronidazole
- Seizure prophylaxis for all patients (e.g., phenytoin)
- Management of increased intracranial pressure may include head elevation, corticosteroids, mannitol, and hyperventilation if intubated
- Surgical debridement, drainage, and culture indicated for a large abscess resulting in a significant mass effect, abscess associated with foreign bodies, or abscess with unknown source of infection
  - Surgical removal is only possible after the abscess has become encapsulated (may take 4–6 weeks)
- The original source of the abscess must be found and appropriately treated

Prognosis/Complications

- Prognosis is excellent when early diagnosis and appropriate treatment are provided
  - If there is little or no dissemination, full recovery occurs in 80% of patients
- Significant neurologic deficits may not be reversible despite appropriate treatment
- Encapsulated abscesses may be removed without neurologic sequelae
- Multiple abscesses must be followed with serial MRIs and IV antimicrobials must be continued for 6 wk
- Long-term seizure disorders may result

SECTION SEVEN

61. Spinal Epidural Abscess

Etiology/Pathophysiology

- Spinal epidural abscess is a surgical emergency
- An infectious mass in the epidural space that compresses the spinal cord
  - The thoracic cord is most likely to be involved, often T4-T8
  - Infection lodges between the dural space and vertebral bone, usually on the dorsal surface
  - May extend along several vertebral segments
- Predisposing factors include skin and soft tissue infections, back injuries, and vertebral osteomyelitis
- Usually spreads hematogenously from remote sites
  - Staphylococcal infections are the most common, usually from the skin
  - Other organisms come from the urinary tract, lungs, heart, and bowel
- Contiguous spread is also common, especially secondary to osteomyelitis in diabetics and intravenous drug users
- Tuberculosis is a frequent cause in developing countries and immunosuppressed patients

Differential Dx

- Subcutaneous paraspinal abscess
- Metastatic spinal tumor
- Intradural tumor (meningioma or neurofibroma)
- Intramedullary spinal tumor
- Acute transverse myelitis
- Disk herniation

Presentation/Signs & Symptoms

- Localized back pain, progressing to radicular pain that radiates around the chest wall
- Fever is usually present, but may be absent or minimal
- Paraparesis
- Ascending paresthesias in the legs
- Flaccidity, followed by spasticity, in the legs
- Urinary retention
- Bilateral Babinski signs

Diagnostic Evaluation

- Initial laboratory studies include CBC with differential (reveals leukocytosis) and ESR (elevated)
- MRI is the ideal imaging modality
  - Reveals isointense lesions on T1 imaging and hyperintense lesions on T2 imaging
- Myelogram may be necessary to visualize the abscess but should be avoided if possible because of the risks of compression of the spinal cord from mass effect

Treatment/Management

- Administer appropriate IV antibiotics
  - IV antibiotics should continue for 6 wk followed by oral antibiotics for 3 mo
  - If there is osseus involvement (i.e., osteomyelitis), antitubercular drugs should be instituted until the etiology is confirmed by cultures
- IV corticosteroids should be administered to reduce spinal cord edema
- Laminectomy and decompression with drainage of abscess is indicated in all cases
  - An anterior approach may be necessary if the vertebral body is involved

Prognosis/Complications

- Prognosis is good if surgical relief is begun within hours
- Residual paraparesis occurs in the majority of cases

62. Fungal & Tubercular Infections

Etiology/Pathophysiology

- Produce subacute or chronic inflammation of the meninges and brain parenchyma
- Commonly seen in immunocompromised individuals
- Cryptococcus is the most commonly involved fungus, especially in AIDS patients
- Tubercular infections are now rare in western countries
- Primary infections generally occur in the skin, lungs, or joints

Differential Dx

- Aseptic or viral meningitis
- Neoplastic meningitis
- Encephalitis
- Bacterial meningitis, especially *Listeria monocytogenes*
- Sarcoid meningitis
- Toxoplasmosis of the brain in AIDS patients
- Spongiform encephalopathies

Presentation/Signs & Symptoms

- Tuberculous meningitis and fungal meningitis are commonly confused, but TB infections tend to be more severe, have a more rapid course (weeks versus months), and generally are more febrile
- Headache
- Fever
- Confusion and subacute dementia
- Gait disturbances
- Cranial neuropathies, especially with TB (e.g., third or sixth cranial nerve palsy)
- Nausea/vomiting
- Personality changes
- Seizures
- Meningismus

Diagnostic Evaluation

- Laboratory studies may include CBC with differential, chemistries, blood cultures, and chest X-ray or chest CT
- Head CT or MRI reveals meningeal enhancement and possibly hydrocephalus or fungal/tubercular abscesses
- Lumbar puncture with CSF analysis is always abnormal
  - Findings in fungal disease include lymphocytic pleocytosis (few cells to several hundred), low glucose, elevated protein, and elevated opening pressure
  - Fungal cultures take weeks to grow, but cryptococcal antigen is present in about 90% of cases
  - Findings in TB reveal pleocytosis (20–500 cells, mostly lymphocytes; however, PMNs may predominate in immunocompromised patients), high protein, low glucose
  - Acid-fast bacilli stain is positive in 25% of cases and culture is positive in 60% of cases; PCR for mycobacteria DNA has high sensitivity and specificity
  - CSF complement-fixing antibodies may identify fungi

Treatment/Management

- Administer appropriate antimicrobial agents
- Tubercular meningitis is treated with three antimicrobials for 6 mo followed by two agents for 4 additional months
  - Medications include isoniazid, rifampin, ethambutol, pyrazinamide, or streptomycin
- Antifungal therapy includes IV amphotericin B and oral flucytosine for 6 wk

Prognosis/Complications

- Mortality for TB meningitis is 10% in immunocompromised patients and 20% in AIDS patients
- 20–30% of cases have resultant neurologic sequelae including normal pressure hydrocephalus with dementia, seizures, and cranial nerve dysfunction (e.g., third, sixth, and eighth cranial nerve palsy)
- Fungal infections may be chronic despite treatment, with 10% relapse
- Mortality from cryptococcal meningitis may be as high as 40%, despite therapy
- Complications include normal pressure hydrocephalus, dementia, and multiple cranial neuropathies

63. Spongiform Encephalopathy/Prion Diseases

Etiology/Pathophysiology

- This group of disorders is referred to as spongiform encephalopathies, as there are small holes created in the brain
- Spongiform encephalopathies caused by an abnormal, infectious protein
  - Unlike other infectious agents (e.g., viruses, bacteria), proteins do not contain nucleic acids
- The associated syndromes include a long latency period (years) followed by dementia, gait disturbances and ataxia, visual disturbances, and myclonus, leading to death in less than a year
- Disease may be inherited, acquired, or sporadic
  - Familial types include familial Creutzfelt-Jakob disease (CJD), Gerstmann-Straussler-Scheinker disease, and fatal familial insomnia
  - Sporadic CJD is most the most common prion disease, occurring in 1 per million people; caused by reconfiguration of the patient's own prion protein (prp)
  - Acquired disease may be iatrogenic from neurosurgical procedures, corneal transplants, or human growth hormone administration; kuru was formerly seen in New Guinea due to cannibalistic practices
- There is concern about new-variant CJD, possibly from bovine spongiform encephalopathy ("mad cow disease"), primarily in England

Differential Dx

- Alzheimer's disease
- Pick's disease
- Other CNS infections (herpes simplex encephalitis, fungal or tubercular meningitis)
- Wernicke's encephalopathy
- Lewy body disease
- Parkinson's disease
- Drug intoxications (e.g., lithium)
- Progressive supranuclear palsy
- Cortico-basal-ganglionic degeneration
- Metabolic encephalopathy (e.g., uremia, hepatic encephalopathy)

Presentation/Signs & Symptoms

- CJD: Insomnia, agitation, confusion, visual impairment, ataxia, aphasia, myoclonus, rigidity, severe dementia
- New-variant CJD: Personality changes, sensory symptoms (e.g., burning in extremities)
- Fatal familial insomnia: Insomnia is the predominant symptom, autonomic changes (e.g., postural hypotension, or anhidrosis)

Diagnostic Evaluation

- MRI is usually normal but may reveal basal ganglia hypointensities
- EEG typically shows periodic sharp discharges; however, EEG in new-variant CJD is normal
- CSF analysis is normal except for the presence of the 14-3-3 protein, which is a marker for neuronal loss in CJD
- Brain biopsy reveals typical spongiform changes in the parenchyma

Treatment/Management

- There is no cure
- Supportive care may include benzodiazepines (e.g., clonazepam) to treat myoclonus
- Precautions should be taken to avoid direct contact with infected CNS material, including CSF

Prognosis/Complications

- All prion diseases have life expectancy of less than 2 y
  - The average life expectancy in patients with CJD is 8 mo following diagnosis
  - The average life expectancy in patients with new-variant CJD is 16 mo

64. HIV & AIDS

Etiology/Pathophysiology

- HIV causes widespread destruction of the central and peripheral nervous systems both by direct invasion of the virus into the nervous system and by immunosuppression, which allows opportunistic infections as result of impaired cellular immunity
    - Direct insults include brain atrophy, meningoencephalitis, vacuolar myopathy, peripheral neuropathy, and myopathy
    - Consequences of impaired cellular immunity include lymphoma of the brain (5% of AIDS patients), neurosyphilis, viral infections of the nervous system (including progressive multifocal leukoencephalopathy (PML and CMV), tubercular infections of the nervous system, fungal infections of the nervous system (e.g., cryptococcus), protozoal infections (e.g., toxoplasmosis), and *Nocardia*
- AIDS dementia complex occurs in 25% of patients with advanced disease
- The virus may result in vacuoles and demyelination in the brain and spinal cord

Differential Dx

- Encephalitis
- Dementia of other etiologies
- Multiple sclerosis
- Cerebral neoplasm
- Bacterial or viral meningitis
- Acute transverse myelitis
- Peripheral neuropathy
- Spongiform encephalopathies
- Polymyositis
- Wernicke's encephalopathy

Presentation/Signs & Symptoms

- Brain insults may result in a subcortical-type dementia with personality changes and apathy, but language function remains largely intact; headache, meningismus, fever, seizures, gait disturbances, visual field defects
    - HIV meningoencephalitis may present as aseptic meningitis
- Spinal cord lesions may result in paraplegia and sensory symptoms (e.g., urinary retention)
- Peripheral nerve lesions may result in painful burning extremities, mononeuritis multiplex, and chronic demyelinating polyneuropathy
- Muscle lesions may result in myalgias and proximal paresis

Diagnostic Evaluation

- CD4 counts are usually <100 with CNS involvement
- MRI of brain may show atrophy and white matter demyelinating lesions
    - Toxoplasmosis normally causes ring-enhancing lesions in the basal ganglia areas
    - Lymphoma of brain results in enhancing lesions in the white matter
    - PML results in large demyelinating lesions
    - Meningeal enhancement may be present in meningitis
- CSF reveals increased cells (primarily lymphocytes), elevated protein (in AIDS dementia complex, meningoencephalitis, and cryptococcal meningitis), may have positive cytology, cryptococcal antigen, PCR for Epstein-Barr virus or JC virus, or β-microglobulin
- Slowing of nerve conduction velocities and absent F waves occur in neuropathies
- Toxoplasma titer and serologic test for syphilis

Treatment/Management

- Appropriate antiretroviral therapy as indicated
- Treat opportunistic infections with appropriate antimicrobial or antifungal agents
- AIDS dementia complex is treated with AZT
- CNS lymphoma is treated with brain irradiation
- PML may respond to interferons or cytosine arabinoside
- Polyneuropathy and myopathy are treated symptomatically (e.g., gabapentin, NSAIDs)

Prognosis/Complications

- Prognosis is generally poor if opportunistic infections occur, with mortality within 1 y
- Antiretroviral therapy may preserve life for many years
- CNS lymphoma generally has a poor prognosis, but remissions are possible following brain irradiation
- Opportunistic infections generally have a worse prognosis in AIDS patients
- PML is fatal within 1 y in 90% of cases

Neoplastic/ Paraneoplastic Conditions of the Central Nervous System

LARA J. KUNSCHNER, MD

65. Gliomas

Etiology/Pathophysiology

- An invasive tumor composed of glial cells that may be slow-growing or highly malignant
- Tumors arise from cerebral astrocytes (astrocytoma, glioblastoma multiforme), oligodendrocytes (oligodendroglioma), or neuroectoderm (medulloblastoma)
- Gliomas are graded by cellularity and degree of malignancy
  - Grade I: Subependymal giant cell astrocytoma, pilocytic astrocytoma
  - Grade II: Ependymoma, diffuse astrocytoma, oligodendroglioma, central neurocytoma
  - Grade III: Anaplastic astrocytoma, anaplastic oligodendroglioma, anaplastic ependymoma
  - Grade IV: Glioblastoma multiforme, anaplastic oligodendroglioma/ glioblastoma multiforme
- Low-grade gliomas may recur at a lower or more malignant grade
- The majority of primary malignant brain tumors arise from de novo genetic mutations
- Glioblastoma multiforme is the most common primary brain tumor

Differential Dx

- Medulloblastoma
- Meningioma
- Metastatic tumor
- Brain abscess
- CNS lymphoma
- Unusual infections (e.g., toxoplasmosis)
- Demyelinating disease ("tumoral multiple sclerosis")

Presentation/Signs & Symptoms

- Clinical presentation depends on tumor location and rate of growth
- Low-grade tumors generally present with seizures
- High-grade tumors often present with headache, confusion, focal neurological signs (e.g., arm or leg weakness), with or without seizures
  - The more malignant the tumor, the more rapid the loss of neurologic function
- Nausea/vomiting
- Lethargy

Diagnostic Evaluation

- History and physical exam, including a detailed neurologic examination
- Head CT with and without contrast will identify most cases
- Head MRI with and without gadolinium enhancement is the best imaging modality to define the location and extent of the tumor
- Imaging shows infiltrative mass, poorly defined margins, edema, mass effect
- Pathologic diagnosis for grading based on the degree of cellularity and pleomorphism
  - Heterogeneity within the tumor is common
- Astrocytomas usually are positive with immunostaining for glial fibrillary acidic protein
- Diagnostic features of glioblastoma multiforme include vascular proliferation or coagulative necrosis and may be accompanied by pseudopalisading of neoplastic cells

Treatment/Management

- Steroids should be administered in all cases to decrease peritumoral edema
- Anticonvulsant therapy
- Stereotaxic biopsy and/or open excision when possible; maximal resection may confer survival benefit
- Fractionated radiation therapy may be useful for grade III and IV tumors and possibly grade II
  - Following resection, grade I and II tumors are often followed without radiation
- Chemotherapy is used for anaplastic oligodendrogliomas and may provide modest survival benefits for other tumor types

Prognosis/Complications

- The most important prognostic variables are age at diagnosis, tumor histology, completeness of resection, and functional status
- Survival depends on grade of tumor
  - Grade I: >20 y
  - Grade II: >10 y
  - Grade III: <5 y
  - Grade IV: <3 y
- Radiation therapy may be complicated by radiation necrosis of surrounding brain tissue
  - Dementia is common following radiation
- Chemotherapy is often associated with systemic side effects
- Gliomas are rarely cured by surgery alone, except for grade I tumors

66. Metastatic Brain Tumors

Etiology/Pathophysiology

- A common sequela of malignancies that carries an extremely poor prognosis
- The most common brain tumors, accounting for approximately 150,000 new cases per year in the U.S.
- Incidence is increasing as survival from various systemic cancers improves
- In order of frequency, the most common cancers to metastasize to the brain are lung cancer, breast cancer, malignant melanoma, renal cell carcinoma, and colorectal cancer
    - These account for 85% of all metastatic brain tumors
- 50% of cases result in a solitary mass; the remainder present with two or more tumors simultaneously
- May involve the parenchyma, leptomeninges, or the dura
- Tumors usually arise from hematologic spread from a distant primary source; rarely occur by direct extension from a bony site
- CNS may be a "protected site" from chemotherapies due to the blood-brain barrier that blocks many anticancer treatments from achieving therapeutic levels in the CNS and may be more prone to metastases than other tissues
- Normally associated with significant peritumoral edema and potential for brain herniation

Differential Dx

- Primary CNS tumors (e.g., glioma)
- Meningioma
- Primary CNS lymphoma
- Brain abscess
- Demyelinating disease ("tumoral multiple sclerosis")

Presentation/Signs & Symptoms

- Clinical presentation depends entirely on the location, number of metastases, and rate of tumor growth
- The most common presenting symptom is headache (70–75%)
- Other symptoms include seizures, confusion, hemiparesis, cranial nerve palsy, vomiting, aphasia, visual disturbance, and decreased level of consciousness
- Some patients are initially asymptomatic and the tumor is found upon screening imaging studies at the time of systemic carcinoma diagnosis

Diagnostic Evaluation

- Diagnosis via head CT with and without contrast and MRI
    - Metastatic parenchymal tumors are generally supratentorial, most frequently in the vascular distribution of the middle cerebral arteries, particularly arterial border zones, but may also occur in areas with a poor blood-brain barrier (e.g., pineal gland, choroid plexus, pituitary)
    - Tend to be roughly spherical masses with sharply delineated borders
- A solitary mass in a patient with known systemic cancer is not immediately diagnostic for metastasis; primary CNS tumors, abscess, or meningioma must be ruled out, often with direct biopsy/resection.
- Metastatic workup to identify the primary tumor: Recommended studies include, but are not limited to, chest X-ray and CT, abdominal and pelvic CT, mammogram in women, stool guaiac, bone scan, urinalysis, and hematologic/bone marrow examination for lymphoma

Treatment/Management

- Acute neurologic symptoms should be initially stabilized (control of seizures, steroids for cerebral edema, antiemetics for nausea); in severe cerebral edema with impending herniation, begin emergent intubation for hyperventilation and administration of hyperosmotic agents (e.g., mannitol)
- Tumors are often amenable to surgical resection; surgical removal followed by fractionated radiation therapy (in divided doses to decrease side effects) is used if 2 or fewer lesions present, the primary tumor is known, and no disseminated disease
- Fractionated radiation alone is indicated if disseminated disease or >2 lesions; prevents/delays neurological deficits, may restore function, decreases corticosteroid needs, and may improve survival
- Excisional or stereotaxic radiosurgery are used to treat lesions with an unknown primary tumor

Prognosis/Complications

- Outcome of metastatic tumors primarily depends on control of the primary disease
- Median survival ranges from 4–11 mo, depending on tumor type, systemic cancer status, and number of brain metastases (i.e., one completely resected tumor has longer survival than multiple tumors in a patient with advanced metastatic disease outside the brain)
- Surgical decompression for posterior fossa metastases may be palliative

67. Meningiomas

Etiology/Pathophysiology

- A benign, slow-growing tumor that arises from the meninges
- Occurs in multiple locations, including the spinal cord
- Comprise approximately 20% of primary intracranial tumors
- Arises from arachnoid cap cells around the cerebral veins and sinuses
- Always attached to the dura
- Associated with prior brain irradiation, trauma, and genetic predispositions (e.g., neurofibromatosis type 2)
- Progesterone and estrogen receptors are found in many meningiomas

Differential Dx

- Intraparenchymal tumors
- Metastatic tumor (e.g., prostate) to the skull, dura, or leptomeninges
- Schwannoma
- Brain abscess

Presentation/Signs & Symptoms

- Usually presents with headache, seizures, confusion, and personality changes
- Unique presentations based on location
  - Olfactory groove tumors: Abulic frontal lobe syndrome (apathetic appearance)
  - Sphenoid wing tumors: Unilateral visual loss, headache, seizures
  - Cavernous sinus tumors: Diplopia, facial numbness, headache, decreased visual acuity
  - Parasagittal tumors: Focal motor/ sensory seizures starting in the leg and progressing up the body, arm, and face
  - Convexity tumors: Headache, focal deficits
  - Spinal tumors: Paraparesis, sensory alterations in the lower extremities

Diagnostic Evaluation

- History and neurologic examination
- CT scan shows isodense to slightly hyperdense lesion; may show bony hyperostosis
- MRI shows a well-circumscribed, durally based lesion
  - Lesion is often isointense on T1 weighting, variable on T2
  - "Dural tail" is characteristic
  - Homogeneous tumor enhancement occurs after contrast administration
- Histologic diagnosis may reveal benign, anaplastic, or malignant changes

Treatment/Management

- Anticonvulsant therapy
- Steroid administration for edema
- Observation alone is sufficient in cases where the tumor is not responsible for patient's symptoms (i.e., the tumor was an incidental finding during a neurologic workup for another issue)
- Surgical resection is indicated for symptomatic meningiomas that are amenable to resection; outcomes are best with complete removal and excision of dural attachments
- Radiation therapy may be used as an adjunct to subtotal removal or for recurrences if repeat resection is not feasible

Prognosis/Complications

- Benign meningioma has a 5-y survival rate of >90% and 10-y survival rate of >75%
- Anaplastic meningioma has 5-y survival rate of 50–90%
- Malignant meningioma has 5-y survival rate of 40–60%

68. Acoustic Neuroma/Vestibular Schwannoma

Etiology/Pathophysiology

- A slow-growing neoplasm of cranial nerve VIII
- Begins in the internal auditory canal and may invade the cerebellopontine angle
- Arises from Schwann cells along the vestibular portion of cranial nerve VIII
- These tumors are histologically benign but dangerous because they may compress the brainstem and multiple cranial nerves
- The presence of bilateral acoustic neuromas is diagnostic of neurofibromatosis type 2

Differential Dx

- Meningioma
- Large basilar artery aneurysm
- Epidermoid tumor
- Ménière's disease
- Benign positional vertigo
- Labyrinthitis

Presentation/Signs & Symptoms

- Presenting symptoms include tinnitus, unilateral hearing loss, and/or disequilibrium
- Late symptoms may include facial numbness or weakness of the face
- Hearing loss ranges from mild, high-frequency loss to complete deafness
- Depressed corneal reflex
- Gaze-evoked nystagmus
- Ataxia

Diagnostic Evaluation

- History and neurologic examination with particular attention to hearing loss and tinnitus
- Audiogram to evaluate hearing loss
- CT with contrast or MRI demonstrates enhancing mass in the cerebellopontine angle
  - The intracanalicular component may be visible early on MRI prior to extension to the cerebellopontine angle
- Brainstem auditory evoked responses
- Spinal fluid analysis is not generally indicated but will reveal elevated protein

Treatment/Management

- Watchful waiting is sufficient in select patients as long dormancy periods are common and in general there is a very slow average growth rate
- Microsurgical resection is indicated for tumors larger than 2.5 cm in diameter
- Radiosurgery may be used for tumors under 3 cm

Prognosis/Complications

- 90–100% cure rate with surgical resection
- There is a high rate of unilateral hearing loss with or without facial nerve dysfunction in postoperative patients
- Radiosurgery for tumor "control" may be sufficient in >90% of patients, resulting in less hearing loss

69. Meningeal Carcinomatosis

Etiology/Pathophysiology

- Seeding of the meninges with metastatic cancer
- Develops in up to 5–10% of cancer patients
- Results in infiltration of tumor cells in the cranial nerves and nerve roots throughout the neuraxis; frequently obstructs the flow of spinal fluid resulting in hydrocephalus
- Most commonly seen in leukemia/lymphoma, glioma, medulloblastoma, and breast and lung cancers
- Largely felt to occur secondary to hematogenous spread of the tumor to the leptomeninges
- Rarely due to direct extension from bony metastases
- May be from direct extension into the pia arachnoid by gliomas or medulloblastomas

Differential Dx

- Infectious meningitis
- Inflammatory meningoencephalitis/myelitis
- Paraneoplastic encephalomyelitis
- Cerebrovascular disorders
- Metabolic/nutritional encephalopathies
- Gliomatosis cerebri

Presentation/Signs & Symptoms

- Headache
- Mental status changes
- Nausea/vomiting
- Seizures
- Confusion
- Aphasia
- Cranial nerve dysfunction (e.g., hearing loss, visual loss, facial numbness, vertigo)
- Meningismus
- Papilledema
- Gait disequilibrium
- Focal weakness
- Segmental sensory deficits
- Cauda equina syndrome is common

Diagnostic Evaluation

- History and neurologic examination
- Craniospinal MRI with gadolinium enhancement to evaluate for bulky leptomeningeal deposits or meningeal enhancement
- Head CT is much less sensitive than MRI
- CSF analysis with positive cytology is diagnostic
  - Cytology is positive in 60% of cases on the first tap; however, repeat spinal fluid analysis may be necessary to identify positive cytology
  - Opening pressure measurement is elevated in 50% of cases
  - Cell count >4 in 60–75% of cases
  - Protein >50 mg/dL in 80% of cases
  - Glucose <40 in 40–50% of cases

Treatment/Management

- Treatment options include craniospinal irradiation, intrathecal chemotherapy, and high-dose systemic chemotherapy (methotrexate)
- Due to the high incidence of obstruction of spinal fluid flow, an Ommaya reservoir may be necessary to infuse chemotherapy directly into the ventricles
- Steroid administration may be indicated to reduce edema
- Anticonvulsant therapy

Prognosis/Complications

- If diagnosed in the setting of a poorly controlled solid tumor, there is an extremely poor short-term survival
- If an isolated recurrence of a leukemia or lymphoma, the prognosis is guarded but better than above
- If medulloblastoma is diagnosed, overall survival is 1–3 y

70. Skull Base Tumors

Etiology/Pathophysiology

- The most common types of skull based malignancies are metastatic tumors from distant sites that spread hematogenously to the skull base
  - Most commonly breast, lung, prostate, and myeloma
- Contiguous spread of head and neck tumors may also result in skull base cancers
  - Most common include nasopharyngeal carcinoma, squamous cell carcinoma, osteosarcomas, glomus jugulare tumors, and chordomas that extend to skull base
- There are also many benign tumors that may involve the skull base (e.g., meningioma)
- Carcinomas may erode the skull base foramina and therefore involve the cranial nerves as they exit the skull

Differential Dx

- Meningeal carcinomatosis
- Meningitis (chronic)
- Multiple sclerosis
- Guillain-Barré syndrome
- Sarcoidosis
- Bell's palsy
- Trigeminal neuralgia

Presentation/Signs & Symptoms

- Tumors of the orbit: Proptosis
- Tumors of superior orbital fissure: Ophthalmoparesis
- Tumors of petrous bone: Facial paresis
- Tumors of foramen rotundum: Facial numbness
- Tumors of petrous bone or foramen ovale: Facial pain
- Tumors of foramen jugulare: Hoarseness and dysphagia
- Tumors of hypoglossal foramen: Tongue paralysis and deviation
- Dysarthria may occur with tumors of various areas
- "Numb chin syndrome" occurs due to marrow infiltration of the mandible

Diagnostic Evaluation

- Skull base CT is the most useful diagnostic test to evaluate for erosion of the skull base foramina
- Bone scan
- MRI of brain with contrast
- CSF analysis with cytology to exclude meningeal carcinomatosis

Treatment/Management

- Fractionated local radiation therapy to the skull base is the most effective treatment
- Chemotherapy may be useful to treat the primary cancer
- Pain control with narcotics is usually necessary

Prognosis/Complications

- Prognosis largely depends on control of the primary cancer
- Radiation therapy may relieve pain
- Prognosis is generally poor due to underlying disease and involvement of swallowing resulting in aspiration and death

71. Pituitary Tumors

Etiology/Pathophysiology

- Pituitary adenomas are nearly always benign
- Account for 10–15% of intracranial neoplasms
- Tumors may be secretory (75%) or nonsecretory (25%) of prolactin
- May develop from an intrinsic pituitary neoplastic process or through excess trophic stimulation from the hypothalamus
- Tumors are broadly classified into microadenomas (<1 cm) versus macroadenomas (>1 cm)
- The most common histologic type is chromophobic adenoma

Differential Dx

- Pituitary carcinoma
- Craniopharyngioma
- Meningioma
- Germ cell tumor
- Chordoma
- Glioma
- Metastatic tumor
- Inflammatory conditions (e.g., sarcoidosis, histiocytosis)
- Giant aneurysm
- Rathke pouch cyst
- Empty sella syndrome

Presentation/Signs & Symptoms

- Presenting symptoms occur due to endocrine manifestations of hormonal excess (amenorrhea, galactorrhea, acromegaly, Cushing's disease, secondary hyper-thyroidism), hormonal deficiency (in cases of chromophobic adenomas resulting in panhypopituitarism) or compression of the optic chiasm (visual field defects, headache)
- Rarely, pituitary apoplexy (infarction) may occur, resulting in panhypopituitarism and blindness

Diagnostic Evaluation

- MRI may demonstrate a sellar mass with possible suprasellar extension and pituitary stalk deviation
    - MRI identifies only 70% of microadenomas
    - Macroadenomas may show diffuse sellar enlargement or destruction
- Initial endocrine evaluation includes prolactin, growth hormone, ACTH, LH, FSH, TSH, thyroxine, cortisol, insulin-like growth factor-1 (IGF-1), testosterone, and estradiol levels

Treatment/Management

- Hormonal/receptor pharmacotherapy (e.g., dopamine agonists, somatostatin analogs) is the primary treatment
    - Prolactinomas are treated with dopaminergic agonists (e.g., cabergoline, pergolide, bromocriptine)
- Surgical resection is reserved for tumors that threaten the visual pathways; many cases can be approached transsphenoidally
- Radiotherapy for recurrent or resistant adenomas
- Hormone replacement therapy for pituitary hormone deficiency and panhypopituitarism

Prognosis/Complications

- Most cases result in long-term survival or cure
- Remission with dopamine agonists alone occurs in 70–100% of prolactinomas
- Remission after surgery for acromegaly or Cushing's disease secondary to adenoma is 80–90%

72. Spinal Tumors

Etiology/Pathophysiology

- Spinal tumors may be extradural (metastatic to bone with subsequent collapse and compression of the spinal cord), extramedullary intradural (outside the spinal cord but within the dura), or intramedullary (within the spinal cord)
- Intramedullary tumors are very slow growing but difficult to manage due to their inaccessible location
    - Astrocytoma (low- or high-grade)
    - Ependymoma
    - Ganglioglioma
    - Primitive neuroectodermal tumors (PNET)
- Extramedullary intradural tumors arise from the dura or meninges and carry a better prognosis because they are more accessible
    - Meningioma
    - Neurofibroma
    - Metastatic tumors (85% extend from vertebral body tumor)
- Extradural tumors are almost exclusively secondary metastatic solid cancers or lymphoma and carry a poor prognosis

Differential Dx

- Spinal epidural abscess
- Herpes zoster infection
- Acute transverse myelitis
- Spondylotic myelopathy
- Syringomyelia
- Radiation myelitis

Presentation/Signs & Symptoms

- Intramedullary tumors commonly present with nonspecific back pain (worse in recumbent position), mild sensory complaints, subtle gait disturbance, leg weakness, and urinary retention
- Extramedullary intradural tumors generally present with thoracic radicular pain, ascending paresthesias in the legs, urinary retention, and spastic paraparesis
- Extradural symptoms include severe bony pain and point tenderness, paraparesis, and ascending paresthesias in the legs with urinary retention

Diagnostic Evaluation

- Plain films may show spinal canal enlargement, pedicle erosion, scoliosis in children, or may be normal in adults
- MRI with gadolinium enhancement is diagnostic
- CT myelography is rarely necessary but is used if MRI is contraindicated

Treatment/Management

- Corticosteroid administration if significant cord edema is present
- Radiotherapy for extradural metastases is usually sufficient
- Surgical resection is indicated for accessible extramedullary and intradural tumors
- Radiotherapy and chemotherapy have a limited role for intramedullary tumors

Prognosis/Complications

- Extradural metastatic tumors generally present with advanced systemic malignancy; these carry the worst prognosis and overall survival is related to the systemic malignancy
- Neurological prognosis depends on function at time of initial intervention
- Prognosis in cases of cord compression related to the severity and duration of the compression
- Low-grade intramedullary tumors have favorable prognosis if the tumor can be completely resected
- Malignant intramedullary tumors generally carry a poor survival (<18–24 mo), depending on histology and resectability of the tumor

73. Paraneoplastic Conditions

Etiology/Pathophysiology

- A group of neurologic disorders related to autoimmune damage to the nervous system by tumor antigens; symptoms are not caused by immediate tissue destruction, invasion, or metastasis by a tumor
- Syndromes are usually antibody-mediated
- Commonly associated with small cell carcinoma and gynecologic cancers
- Limbic/bulbar encephalitis: Inflammatory disorder involving the mesial temporal lobe structures
- Subacute sensory neuropathy: A painful neuropathy with distal and proximal sensory loss usually due anti-Hu antibody
- Cerebellar degeneration: Subacute ataxia and atrophy of the cerebellum associated with anti-Yo antibodies
- Lambert-Eaton myasthenic syndrome: Proximal fatigable weakness and autonomic symptoms (e.g., dry mouth) associated with anti-voltage gated calcium channel antibodies
- Opsoclonus/myoclonus: Ocular movement disorders and ataxia associated with anti-Ri antibodies
- Dermatomyositis/polymyositis: Seen primarily in males with lung cancer; no specific antibody identified; associated with proximal muscle weakness
- Stiff person syndrome: Rigidity and muscle spasms associated with anti-glutamic acid dehydrogenase antibody; primarily related to breast cancer

Differential Dx

- Metastatic disease
- Nutritional or metabolic disorders
- Infectious disease (e.g., encephalitis, meningitis)
- Degenerative disorders
- Neurotoxicity secondary to cancer treatments

Presentation/Signs & Symptoms

- Limbic/bulbar encephalitis: Confusion, agitation, anxiety, depression, seizures, hallucinations, and acute dementia
- Subacute sensory neuropathy: Pain, paresthesias, and sensory ataxia
- Cerebellar degeneration: Ataxia, dysarthria, and disequilibrium
- Lambert-Eaton myasthenic syndrome: Proximal muscular aching and weakness that may improve with exercise
- Opsoclonus/myoclonus: Ataxia and jerking of the eyes in multiple directions
- Dermatomyositis/polymyositis: Heliotropic rash, proximal muscle weakness
- Stiff person syndrome presents as rigidity of muscles

Diagnostic Evaluation

- EMG/nerve conduction studies for neuropathy or weakness
- MRI with gadolinium of brain and/or spinal cord if symptoms suggest a central localization
- Serum and CSF analysis for paraneoplastic antibodies
  - Anti-Hu (small cell lung cancer): Sensory neuropathy, encephalomyelitis, cerebellar degeneration
  - Anti-CV-2 (small cell lung cancer): Sensory neuropathy, limbic encephalitis
  - Anti-Yo (breast/gynecologic cancers): Cerebellar degeneration
  - Anti-Ri (breast, lung, GI cancers): Opsoclonus/myoclonus
  - Anti-Ma-Ta (testicular cancer): Limbic encephalitis, cerebellar degeneration
  - Anti-voltage gated calcium receptor (small cell lung cancer): Myasthenic syndrome
  - Anti-Jo-1 (several cancers): Polymyositis/dermatomyositis

Treatment/Management

- Control of the primary malignancy may arrest progression of neurological symptoms, but may not improve the symptoms
- Plasma exchange/IVIG have been used based on anecdotal reports of symptomatic improvement
- High-dose corticosteroids are of questionable benefit

Prognosis/Complications

- Overall survival is determined by the primary malignancy
- Neurological functioning rarely recovers substantially, but may plateau with treatment

Degenerative & Metabolic Disorders

DAVID G. WRIGHT, MD

74. Alcoholism

Etiology/Pathophysiology

- Disorders of the CNS and PNS occur due to direct toxic effects of alcohol and secondary vitamin deficiencies
- Intoxication syndromes include drunkenness, "blackouts," and coma
- Withdrawal syndromes include seizures and delirium tremens
- Nutritional deficiencies include alcoholic neuropathy and Wernicke-Korsakoff syndrome
  - Wernicke-Korsakoff syndrome is a disorder characterized by confusion, ophthalmoparesis, nystagmus, and ataxia with or without peripheral neuropathy with damage to regions of the thalamus and periaqueductal gray matter due to thiamine deficiency
- Acute and chronic hepatic encephalopathy may occur secondary to liver failure
- Direct alcoholic toxicity may cause cerebellar atrophy

Differential Dx

- Medication intoxication (e.g., dilantin, benzodiazepines)
- Medication withdrawal syndromes (e.g., barbiturates, benzodiazepines)
- Ataxia or encephalopathy due to medical conditions unrelated to alcoholism
- Traumatic injuries to the nervous system
- Other causes of neuropathy (e.g., diabetes mellitus, neoplasm)
- Multiple sclerosis
- Paraneoplastic cerebellar degeneration
- Multiple system atrophy

Presentation/Signs & Symptoms

- Deterioration in interpersonal relations, physical health, and occupation
- Blackouts of memory, irresponsible behavior, physical injury, or stupor and coma during periods of intoxication
- Tremulousness, agitation, delirium with hallucinations, or seizures during periods of withdrawal
- Chronic ataxia, memory loss, or dementia associated with nutritional deficiency
- Cerebellar atrophy may result in ataxia, dysarthria, and disequilibrium

Diagnostic Evaluation

- History and physical examination
- Brain imaging may be indicated to evaluate for traumatic complications of intoxication, especially subdural hematoma, and may also detect cerebellar atrophy
- EEG in patients with seizures or encephalopathy (triphasic waves are seen in patients with hepatic encephalopathy)
- Nerve conduction studies to evaluate peripheral neuropathy
- Initial laboratory studies include CBC with differential, blood ammonia level, LFTs, vitamin B_{12} and folate levels
- Psychiatric evaluation for underlying depression

Treatment/Management

- Detoxification including prophylaxis for delirium tremens followed by addiction counseling (e.g., Alcoholics Anonymous)
- Withdrawal seizures are usually not treated unless they are prolonged or recurrent, or a focally abnormal EEG with focal brain pathology is present
- Delirium should be managed in an ICU setting with frequent, small doses of short-acting benzodiazepines and IV fluids
- Nutritional deficiencies should be aggressively corrected with B-complex vitamins and parenteral thiamine
  - Thiamine must be administered prior to IV fluids or glucose repletion to prevent acute Wernicke's encephalopathy with coma

Prognosis/Complications

- Delirium tremens carries a 5% mortality
- Increased risk of suicide
- About 1/3 of patients achieve sobriety with strong encouragement of physician, family, and addiction programs

75. Vitamin Deficiencies

Etiology/Pathophysiology

- Subacute combined degeneration of the spinal cord: Demyelination of the lateral and posterior columns of the spinal cord due to impaired absorption of vitamin B_{12} secondary to lack of intrinsic factor
- Wernicke-Korsakoff syndrome: Symmetrical hemorrhagic necrosis with neuronal damage, demyelination, and astrocytosis in bilateral thalamus, cerebellar vermis, and periaqueductal gray matter of the midbrain due to vitamin B_1 deficiency, most commonly in alcoholics
- Nutritional polyneuropathy: Primarily results in axonal damage due to deficiency in multiple B vitamins and associated with malnutrition; also most common in alcoholics
- Bariatric surgery for weight reduction may result in thiamine and vitamin B_{12} deficiency

Differential Dx

- Subacute combined degeneration: Other forms of sensory ataxia, tabes dorsalis, diabetes mellitus
- Wernicke-Korsakoff syndrome: Posterior circulation ischemic stroke, posterior fossa neoplasm with obstructive hydrocephalus
- Nutritional polyneuropathy: Other causes of axonal neuropathy, mostly toxic and metabolic

Presentation/Signs & Symptoms

- Subacute combined degeneration: Paresthesias followed by sensory ataxia, progressive weakness in legs, and variable psychiatric symptoms; vibratory and position sense are lost prior to pain and temperature sense; megaloblastic anemia may be present
- Wernicke-Korsakoff syndrome: Truncal ataxia, ophthalmoplegia, and short-term memory loss
- Nutritional polyneuropathy: Paresthesias, burning feet, weakness including foot drop, and sensory ataxia
- Vitamin B_{12} deficiency may cause isolated polyneuropathy or dementia

Diagnostic Evaluation

- Subacute combined degeneration:
  - Laboratory findings include low vitamin B_{12} level and elevated homocysteine and methylmalonic acid levels
  - Presence of anti-parietal cell antibody, anti-intrinsic factor antibody
  - Schilling test to evaluate for the presence of intrinsic factor
- Wernicke-Korsakoff syndrome and nutritional polyneuropathy:
  - Diagnosis is based on history and physical examination and confirmed by response to treatment
  - EMG may show significant decrease in amplitude and mild-to-moderate slowing in nerve conductions

Treatment/Management

- Vitamin B_{12} deficiency and subacute combined degeneration: Intramuscular vitamin B_{12} administration twice weekly for 2 wk, then weekly for 3 mo, then monthly
- Wernicke-Korsakoff syndrome: Parenteral thiamine (vitamin B_1) administration daily for 3 d followed by oral supplementation with B-complex vitamins
  - Always administer thiamine prior to IV glucose to prevent acute exacerbation of Wernicke's syndrome
- Nutritional polyneuropathy: Well-balanced diet plus multivitamin supplementation with B-complex vitamins

Prognosis/Complications

- With prompt treatment, most acquired deficits are reversible over weeks to months
- Untreated B_{12} deficiency and B_1 deficiency lead to irreversible CNS damage, dementia, and inability to ambulate
- Untreated polyneuropathy may result in disability due to multifocal motor neuropathy and, in severe cases, cardiomyopathy

76. Alzheimer's Disease

Etiology/Pathophysiology

- A common, relentlessly progressive form of dementia usually seen in advanced years, characterized by personality change, language dysfunction, and memory failure
- Comprises at least 50% of all cases of dementia
- Characterized by atrophy of the cerebral cortex, particularly the temporal lobes
- Neuronal loss primarily affects cholinergic neurons; associated with 50–90% reduction in choline acetyltransferase activity
- Primarily affects elderly patients; however, there is a familial form that affects younger patients
- Prevalence <1% under age 65; 30–40% of age 85 and older
- Genetic mutations have been implicated, such as apoE e4 polymorphism of the apolipoprotein gene on chromosome 19
- Histology shows neurofibrillary tangles (filaments with tau protein), neuritic plaques (core of extracellular amyloid), and granular-vacuolar degeneration

Differential Dx

- Normal cognitive aging
- Pseudodementia of depression
- Other dementing diseases (e.g., multi-infarct dementia, Pick's or Parkinson's disease, progressive supranuclear palsy, diffuse Lewy body disease, NPH)
- Metabolic and endocrine disorders (e.g., vitamin B_{12} deficiency, Wernicke's encephalopathy)
- Medication effects
- Infections (e.g., HIV, CJD, neurosyphilis, cryptococcal meningitis)

Presentation/Signs & Symptoms

- Normal consciousness is preserved
- Insidious onset of slowly progressive memory loss
- Later impairment of intellect, language, and abstract thought
- Aphasia, agnosia, and apraxia
- Loss of executive function
- Delusions and hallucinations in 20–40%
- Depression in 25%
- Extrapyramidal symptoms (rigidity, bradykinesia, or postural instability) in 60%
- Seizures in 10–20%
- Myoclonus in 10%

Diagnostic Evaluation

- History and neurologic examination including serial mental status exams and neuropsychological tests
- Definitive diagnosis can only be proven by autopsy: Neurofibrillary tangles and neuritic plaques are seen on microscopic examination
- No laboratory tests or imaging is diagnostic
- Useful tests include head CT scan or MRI (atrophy), EEG (generalized slowing), metabolic profile, thyroid function testing, vitamin B_{12} level, RPR
- Genetic testing for the apo-ε allele may identify familial cases
- CSF analysis may be indicated to exclude infectious etiologies of dementia

Treatment/Management

- There is no cure—treatment is palliative
- Eliminate all unnecessary medications, especially those with known CNS and anticholinergic effects
- Anticholinesterase inhibitors may initially slow progression of the disease (e.g., donepezil, galantamine, rivastigmine)
- NMDA receptor antagonists (memantine) is now being used
- In select cases, SSRIs and neuroleptics (e.g., seroquel, risperdal) may be tried
- Home health support and counseling for caregiver

Prognosis/Complications

- Progressive clinical course with occasional plateaus
- Duration 4–8 y, rarely as long as 20 y (mean time from diagnosis to death is 8 y)
- Eventual terminal state with mutism, incontinence, and limb contractures
- Death most often occurs due to pneumonia

SECTION NINE

77. Multi-Infarct Dementia

Etiology/Pathophysiology

- A common form of dementia that occurs due to multiple large cortical infarctions or subcortical leukoaeriosis (softening of white matter) secondary to multiple, small lacunar infarcts
- Vascular dementia represents 15–30% of dementia patients, the second most common cause of dementia after Alzheimer's disease
- Occurs as a result of generalized arteriosclerosis, most commonly related to hypertension
- If subcortical periventricular and confluent leukoaeriosis accompanies dementia, may be termed Binswanger's disease
- A rare hereditary form in patients ages 20–50 exists, cerebral autosomal-dominant arteriopathy with subcortical infarcts and leukoencephalopathy (CADASIL), which has been linked to chromosome 19

Differential Dx

- Other forms of subcortical dementia (e.g., Lewy body dementia)
- Multiple sclerosis with dementia
- Acute demyelinating encephalomyelitis (ADEM)
- General paresis form of tertiary syphilis
- Normal pressure hydrocephalus

Presentation/Signs & Symptoms

- Symptoms depend on location of strokes
- Cognitive slowing, memory impairment, and pseudobulbar affect (e.g., unprovoked crying or laughing) are seen with multiple lacunar infarctions
- Aphasia, apraxia, and visual spatial impairments are seen in patients with cortical infarcts
- Course is characterized by stepwise worsening as further ischemic attacks occur rather than a progressive decline

Diagnostic Evaluation

- History and physical examination
- Evaluation of stroke risk factors, especially hypertension and cardiac sources of stroke
- Neuropsychiatric evaluation is helpful
- CT and MRI to document infarcts and leukoaeriosis

Treatment/Management

- Aggressive correction of stroke risk factors, including hypertension, hyperlipidemia, and smoking
- Prevention of cardiac embolic stroke with warfarin, especially in patients with A-fib or MI
- Antiplatelet therapy (aspirin or clopidogrel) for stroke prevention
- Acetylcholinesterases (e.g., donepezil, galantamine) may be helpful

Prognosis/Complications

- Shorter survival than in Alzheimer's patients
- Death most commonly occurs due to vascular causes (stroke, MI)

78. Pick's Disease

Etiology/Pathophysiology

- A neuronal degenerative disease that results in severe dementia that primarily involves the temporal lobes
- Frontotemporal lobar atrophy occurs with loss of neurons in the outer layers of the cerebral cortex, astrocytosis, and spongy changes in the neurons
- Idiopathic etiology but familial predisposition exists
- Swollen neurons are present, some with argentophilic inclusions (Pick bodies), which are filaments made up of tau protein
- Pick bodies are seen in about 1/3 of cases at autopsy

Differential Dx

- Multi-infarct dementia
- Alzheimer's dementia
- Normal pressure hydrocephalus
- Temporal lobe neoplasm
- Limbic encephalitis
- Alcoholic dementia
- Huntington's disease
- Psychiatric illnesses (e.g., major depression with psychosis or personality disorders)

Presentation/Signs & Symptoms

- Aphasia and apraxia occur early in 2/3 of cases
- Personality change and socially unacceptable behavior are prominent in most cases
- Frontal signs of abulia and disinterest in personal hygiene
- Signs of limbic dysfunction, such as bulimia and sexual preoccupation

Diagnostic Evaluation

- History and physical examination
- No laboratory test or imaging is diagnostic
- CT scan or MRI may demonstrate frontotemporal atrophy, often unilateral

Treatment/Management

- No treatment to slow dementia except those used in Alzheimer's disease (e.g., donepezil, memantine)
- Social service and psychiatric intervention may be needed for behavioral issues

Prognosis/Complications

- Progressive clinical deterioration in 2–5 y to terminal dementia in a vegetative state

79. Lewy Body Dementia

Etiology/Pathophysiology

- A form of subcortical dementia that presents with frequent hallucinations
- Neuronal degenerative disease with clinical features of Alzheimer's disease and Parkinson's disease
- Prominent finding of Lewy bodies in the cerebral cortex and brainstem (also in pigmented nuclei) at autopsy
- Few neurofibrillary tangles and senile plaques are found (compared to significant numbers in Alzheimer's dementia)

Differential Dx

- Normal cognitive aging
- Pseudodementia of depression
- Other dementias (Alzheimer's disease, multi-infarct dementia, Pick's disease, Parkinson's disease, progressive supranuclear palsy, diffuse Lewy body disease, NPH)
- Metabolic/endocrine disorders (vitamin B_{12} deficiency, Wernicke's encephalopathy)
- Medication effects
- Infections (e.g., HIV, CJD, neurosyphilis, cryptococcal meningitis)

Presentation/Signs & Symptoms

- Cognitive decline is usually the first symptom
- Extrapyramidal movement disorders (parkinsonism) occur later
- Delusions and hallucinations are common and limit the usefulness of antiparkinsonian medications

Diagnostic Evaluation

- History and physical examination; diagnosis is based on clinical presentation
- No laboratory test or imaging is diagnostic
- CT or MRI may reveal cortical atrophy

Treatment/Management

- There is no useful treatment
- Acetylcholinesterase medications may be used but are not very effective
- Judicious use of neuroleptics with the fewest extrapyramidal effects (e.g., risperdal, seroquel)
- Low dose carbidopa/levodopa may improve rigidity

Prognosis/Complications

- Progressive clinical deterioration to a terminally demented state

80. Frontotemporal Dementia

Etiology/Pathophysiology

- A disorder of neuronal degeneration that is often confused with Alzheimer's disease and accounts for 10% of cases of dementia
- Atrophy occurs in the frontal and anterior temporal cortex
- Neuronal loss occurs with microvascular change and astrocytosis, but absence of neurofibrillary tangles, senile plaques, and Lewy bodies
- Age of onset is younger than in Alzheimer's disease (mean 54 y)
- Tau-positive ballooned neurons
- Nearly 50% of cases have a hereditary component, which is linked to the tau gene on chromosome 17
- Subtypes include Pick's disease, primary progressive nonfluent aphasia, semantic dementia (fluent aphasia)
- A syndrome exists that results in frontotemporal dementia and Parkinsonism (FTDP-17)

Differential Dx

- Minimal cognitive impairment of old age
- Multi-infarct dementia
- Alzheimer's dementia
- Lewy body dementia
- Normal pressure hydrocephalus
- Temporal lobe neoplasm
- Limbic encephalitis
- Alcoholic dementia
- Huntington's disease
- Psychiatric illnesses (e.g., major depression with psychosis or personality disorders)

Presentation/Signs & Symptoms

- Presents with disorders of language, cognition, and behavior
- Change in personality and behavior especially results in disinhibition, poor judgment, diminished motivation, and altered executive function
- Progressive language disturbance is more prominent than memory loss
- Parkinsonism, including rigidity and shuffling gait

Diagnostic Evaluation

- No laboratory test or imaging is diagnostic
- Patients should be evaluated for treatable causes of dementia (e.g., medication intoxication, subdural hematoma, normal pressure hydrocephalus)
- Diagnosis is based on clinical features that differ from Alzheimer's disease
  - Younger age of onset
  - Disturbance of behavior, judgment, and language out of proportion to memory loss
  - Higher incidence of familial dementia

Treatment/Management

- Treat reversible causes of dementia as necessary
- Anticholinesterases are not useful
- Serotonergic drugs may be of benefit (e.g., fluvoxamine, fluoxetine, sertraline)
- Social service support for caregivers

Prognosis/Complications

- Inexorable progression to a state of dependence and then terminal vegetative state
- Mean duration of 8 y to death

81. Multiple System Atrophy/Striatonigral Degeneration

Etiology/Pathophysiology

- A group of disorders with degeneration of subcortical structures leading to impoverished movements, ataxia, and/or dementia
- Degeneration of neurons in the putamen, caudate, substantia nigra, and pontocerebellar structures
- Absence of neurofibrillary tangles and Lewy bodies
- Loss of intermediolateral horn cells occurs in Shy-Drager syndrome (see *Shy-Drager Syndrome*)

Differential Dx

- Other forms of subcortical dementia
- Parkinson's disease
- Autonomic neuropathy
- Pure Shy-Drager syndrome
- Pure olivopontocerebellar degeneration

Presentation/Signs & Symptoms

- Combined clinical features of Parkinson's disease, autonomic dysfunction, and cerebellar degeneration
  - Flexed posture, akinesia, gait disorder; tremor is seldom present
  - Orthostatic hypotension or Shy-Drager syndrome, urinary incontinence, impotence, decreased sweating
  - Ataxia, pyramidal tract signs (spasticity)

Diagnostic Evaluation

- History and physical examination
- No laboratory test or imaging is diagnostic
- MRI or CT scan may show pontine and cerebellar atrophy and hypodense putamen

Treatment/Management

- Amantadine or low-dose carbidopa/levodopa
- Jobst stockings and abdominal binders, fludrocortisone, and midodrine may be used for orthostasis

Prognosis/Complications

- Almost half of cases result in severe disability within 5 y
- Gradual progression to dementia
- Vegetative state occurs as in Parkinson's disease

Neuromuscular Disorders

Section 10

SANDEEP RANA, MD
GEORGE A. SMALL, MD

82. Amyotrophic Lateral Sclerosis

Etiology/Pathophysiology

- ALS is a motor neuron disease that involves both CNS and PNS and is relentlessly progressive and fatal
- The anterior horn cells in the spinal cord, and cranial nerve nuclei in the brainstem, are affected first, then the entire motor unit degenerates, resulting in muscular atrophy, weakness, and fasciculations; in addition, the lateral columns of the spinal cord degenerate, causing spasticity
- Etiology is unknown, though there are several hypotheses
  - Excitotoxicity: Glutamate is an excitatory neurotransmitter; excess amounts can cause neuronal cell death
  - Viral infection
  - Apoptosis (programmed cell death)
  - Free radicals: Decreased ability of neurons to clear these destructive molecules
  - Autoimmunity
- Genetic predisposition: 5–10% of patients have familial ALS
  - Some of these patients have SOD gene mutation, which can be identified by commercially available blood tests
  - Familial ALS may have a less severe course
- Usually presents in the fifth and sixth decades of life; may present earlier

Differential Dx

- Benign fasciculations
- Degenerative spine disease with myelopathy and radiculopathy
- Multifocal motor neuropathy
- Multiple sclerosis
- Poliomyelitis
- Inclusion body myopathy
- Arnold-Chiari malformation and syringomyelia
- X-linked spinobulbar muscular atrophy
- Hex A deficiency
- HIV/HTLV myelopathy
- Combined system degenerations (e.g., CMT)

Presentation/Signs & Symptoms

- The syndrome begins with focal weakness, which gradually progresses to involve all extremities
- Muscle fasciculations are common, but normally not the initial presentation
- As disease progresses, combination of lower (e.g., muscle atrophy) and upper motor neuron findings (e.g., spasticity, brisk reflexes) become evident
- Bulbar involvement (e.g., dysarthria, dysphagia, tongue atrophy)
- Sensory system is not involved
- Ocular muscles are spared until the late stages of the disease
- Autonomic systems are spared (e.g., bladder, GI function, sexual function)

Diagnostic Evaluation

- There is no specific test that is diagnostic of ALS; workup is aimed at excluding other causes
- Laboratory studies may include CBC, ESR, ANA, rheumatoid factor, thyroid function tests, vitamin B_{12} level, and serum immunofixation electrophoresis
- Serum CK is mildly elevated
- Imaging studies include MRI of the brain and spinal cord (e.g., rule out cervical spondylosis)
- Nerve conduction studies and EMG demonstrate reduction in the number of motor units, fasciculations, and denervation potentials
- In some patients, lumbar puncture, urine heavy metal screen, and hexoaminidase A enzyme assay are indicated
- In patients with familial ALS, a genetic test for the SOD mutation is available
- Muscle biopsy can be used; reveals group fiber atrophy

Treatment/Management

- There is no cure
- Riluzole is the only drug approved for ALS in the U.S.
  - Effect on disease progression is modest; may slow the progression of disease by a few months
  - Monitor LFTs closely; may be hepatotoxic in some
- Symptom management and comfort measures are the mainstays of therapy (e.g., muscle relaxants, antispastic agents, pulmonary toilet)
- Gastrostomy feeding tubes and noninvasive ventilatory support are offered in advanced stages
  - Ventilatory support in the U.S. is an ethical and financial dilemma as it is enormously expensive and patients have low quality of life
- Hospice care to administer palliative measures is appropriate for terminally ill patients

Prognosis/Complications

- Patients usually succumb to the disease by 3–5 y
- Patients can be kept alive indefinitely with use of ventilator and feeding tube, but may lose all ability to communicate (including eye movements)
- Pulmonary complications (e.g., pneumonia, pulmonary embolus, respiratory failure) are common terminal events
- Advance directives should be pursued early in the course of disease

83. Poliomyelitis

Etiology/Pathophysiology

- A highly communicable disease of the anterior horn cells of the spinal cord caused by a neurotropic enterovirus
- Also affects the brainstem nuclei
- Nearly extinct in developed countries due to widespread vaccination
- Prevalent before the 1950s
- Occurs after febrile illness with severe gastroenteritis in children and young adults
- Associated with epidemic outbreaks
- Postpolio syndrome represents late exacerbation of disease

Differential Dx

- Amyotrophic lateral sclerosis
- Guillain-Barré syndrome
- Miller-Fisher syndrome
- Lyme disease
- Botulism
- Myasthenia gravis
- Other motor neuron diseases (e.g., progressive spinal muscular atrophy)
- West Nile virus infection

Presentation/Signs & Symptoms

- Follows a febrile gastroenteritis
- Asymmetrical weakness of extremities and truncal muscles develops over 48 h
- Fasciculations
- Diminished deep tendon reflexes
- Sensory loss is rare
- Urinary retention
- Muscular atrophy after 3 wk
- Bulbar paralysis (e.g., dysphagia, dysarthria, weak palate)
- Respiratory failure due to weakness of the respiratory musculature
- Pyramidal tract findings (e.g., Babinski sign) are rarely present

Diagnostic Evaluation

- MRI of the spinal cord may show hyperintensities or atrophy
- CSF analysis demonstrates pleocytosis of white cells (usually in the hundreds) typical of viral infections
  - The virus may be cultured in spinal fluid, but is rarely isolated
- EMG show fasciculations and neurogenic potentials

Treatment/Management

- Oral and parenteral vaccines are given in all children in developed countries
- Speech therapy for dysphagia
- Respiratory care, including intubation if necessary
  - Vital capacity and negative inspiratory force must be measured frequently
- Orthotics and physical therapy with active and passive range of motion exercises
- Antiviral therapy is not effective

Prognosis/Complications

- Mortality is 5–10% in affected patients
- If the patient survives the acute stage, respiratory and swallowing difficulties generally recover
- Weakness of extremities persists permanently
- Postpolio syndrome is typically mild and self-limited

84. Progressive Spinal Muscular Atrophy

Etiology/Pathophysiology

- A group of progressive disorders that affect the anterior horn cells of the spinal cord, resulting in muscular atrophy
- Most forms of the disease are due to mutations on chromosome 5 and have an autosomal recessive inheritance
    - There are some less common cases of autosomal dominant, X-linked recessive, and sporadic forms of the disease
- Werdnig-Hoffman disease manifests in early infancy (less than 3 mo), resulting in floppy infant syndrome
    - Death usually occurs within a few years
- Kugelberg-Welander disease manifests in childhood or early adolescence
    - Patients become wheelchair-bound and disabled by early adulthood
- Bulbospinal motorneuronopathy (Kennedy's disease) presents in adults
    - X-linked recessive transmission
    - May mimic ALS
    - Bulbar weakness occurs early
    - Limb weakness
    - Tongue and chin fasciculations
    - Testicular atrophy with gynecomastia

Differential Dx

- Muscular dystrophies
- ALS
- Motor neuropathies (e.g., lead poisoning, mononeuritis multiplex)
- Cervical spondylosis

Presentation/Signs & Symptoms

- Usually presents in infancy or early childhood, though some forms may present later in life
- Patients develop slowly progressive weakness
    - Proximal muscle involvement is more common than distal weakness
- Sensory and autonomic systems are not affected

Diagnostic Evaluation

- Serum CK is normal or mildly elevated, but does not reach the high levels seen in muscular dystrophies
- EMG shows neuropathic changes and is useful to differentiate from muscular dystrophies
- Genetic tests are commercially available
- Muscle biopsy shows alterations of the normal checkerboard pattern of type I and type II muscle fibers to a grouped atrophy pattern of the two fiber types

Treatment/Management

- No treatment is available
- Physical and occupational therapy and orthoses

Prognosis/Complications

- Life expectancy depends on the specific type of syndrome
    - Adult-onset disease is more benign than ALS and is consistent with a long life but severe disability
    - Childhood-onset diseases tend to be more progressive and fatal
- Patients with Kugelberg-Welander disease often develop scoliosis and joint contractures
- Recurrent pneumonias are common

85. Charcot-Marie-Tooth Syndrome

Etiology/Pathophysiology

- CMT is the most common of a group of inherited combined system disorders
  - The different types of CMT have heterogeneous genetic defects
  - The predominant inheritance pattern is autosomal dominant, though there are types of CMT that are X-linked and autosomal recessive
- CMT affects peripheral nerves and spinal cord via demyelination or direct axonal injury
  - Depending on the genetic defect, the patient may have demyelinating or axonal neuropathy
- Age of onset is generally in the teenage and young adult years
- Symptoms are slowly progressive, resulting in moderate incapacitation, but is not fatal

Differential Dx

- Nongenetic etiologies of peripheral neuropathy
  - Diabetes mellitus
  - Monoclonal gammopathy
  - Alcoholic neuropathy
  - Vasculitic neuropathy
  - Nutritional causes (e.g., vitamin B_{12} deficiency)
  - Medication-induced neuropathy
- Other inherited neuropathies (e.g., Friedreich's ataxia, Dejerine-Sottas neuropathy, Roussy-Lévy syndrome)

Presentation/Signs & Symptoms

- The syndrome begins with weakness and atrophy of the distal leg muscles
- Foot deformities occur, including high arch (pes cavus) with hammer toes
- Development of physical milestones is usually delayed in childhood cases
- With progression of the disease, weakness spreads to the distal upper extremity muscles
- Deep tendon reflexes are decreased
- There may or may not be associated sensory loss
- There is usually a history of other family members with similar symptoms

Diagnostic Evaluation

- Nerve conduction studies in cases of the classic demyelinating forms of CMT show uniformly slow velocities with prolonged latencies
- Nerve biopsy reveals an "onion bulb" formation
- Genetic tests are now commercially available to identify several common genetic mutations associated with CMT

Treatment/Management

- No specific treatment is available; gene therapy is promising, but research is still in the preliminary stages
- Occupational and physical therapy is the mainstay of treatment
- Ankle-foot orthotic braces are helpful for patients with foot drop
- Genetic counseling is important

Prognosis/Complications

- Most patients with CMT have normal life spans
- With aggressive occupational and physical therapy, patients are able to lead independent and productive lives
- Kyphoscoliosis is common

86. Guillain-Barré Syndrome

Etiology/Pathophysiology

- An autoimmune inflammatory polyneuropathy in which segmental demyelination of the peripheral nerves and nerve roots occur, resulting in reversible weakness and sensory loss
  - The most vulnerable parts of the nerve are the root and its most distal nerve segment, where the blood-nerve barrier is at its weakest
  - Criteria for diagnosis include symmetrical weakness and areflexia occurring over 4–5 wk
  - The attack may be mild, resulting in only ataxia, or severe, with rapid paralysis of bulbar and respiratory muscles
  - Most cases reach a nadir within 2 wk
- Usually preceded (50% of cases) by a viral syndrome or *Campylobacter jejuni* infection; may also follow surgeries or immunizations
- Several theories suggest that an antibody- and complement-mediated attack upon myelin sheaths may be a factor in the development of GBS
- There are many types of GBS; most cases are diseases of demyelination
- Incidence of 1/100,000
- Incidence gradually increases with age, but may occur at any age from infancy to old age

Differential Dx

- Unilateral or bilateral Bell's palsy
- Lyme disease
- HIV disease
- Aseptic meningitis
- Myasthenia gravis
- Botulism
- Tic paralysis
- Acute myopathy
- West Nile virus
- Poliomyelitis
- Chronic immune demyelinating polyneuropathy
- Acute intermittent porphyria

Presentation/Signs & Symptoms

- Initial presentation may include only paresthesias in hands and feet
- Progressive weakness, aching sensation, and/or pain in two or more limbs
  - Weakness is usually symmetrical
  - Often ascends from lower extremities
  - Reaches maximum weakness in 4–5 wk
  - Bilateral facial muscle weakness occurs in 70% of patients
  - Extraocular, swallowing, and respiratory muscles may be affected
- Reflexes are diminished or absent
- Autonomic symptoms may occur (e.g., SVT, heart block, severe swings in BP)
- Sensory loss including vibration and position sense common

Diagnostic Evaluation

- EMG is nonspecific and may be normal in the first few weeks of disease; reveals motor units that are recruited in a reduced or irregular fashion
- Characteristic nerve conduction study abnormalities are strongly suggestive of the diagnosis: The most common abnormalities include dispersion or absence of F responses, prolonged distal latencies, and conduction block
- CSF analysis reveals albumino-cytologic dissociation (elevated protein with relatively normal cell counts)
  - Up to 10 lymphocytes may be present in normal individuals and up to 50 lymphocytes in HIV patients
- Immunologic tests provide only supportive data
- Findings that mitigate against diagnosis of GBS: Thoracic sensory level involvement, persisting bowel or bladder defects, monoparesis, purely sensory symptoms, presence of upper motor neuron signs

Treatment/Management

- Recognition of respiratory status is the most important initial management issue
  - Negative inspiratory force and vital capacity can be done at the bedside
  - When vital capacity falls below 15–20 cc/kg (normal 65 cc/kg), V/Q mismatching occurs and intubation may be necessary
- Patients who cannot walk or have abnormal respiratory parameters require inpatient care in a monitored setting; should be treated with IVIG or plasmapheresis; administer IVIG/plasmapheresis over 5 d within 2 wk of symptom onset
- Anticoagulation for DVT prophylaxis
- Frequent BP checks are necessary as myelinated segments of autonomic nerves can be affected causing rapid swings in BP with increased mortality
- Steroids are ineffective

Prognosis/Complications

- Prognosis for walking at 6 mo or improving at least one grade on the MRC scale is dramatically improved in patients receiving IVIG or plasma exchange
- 90% of patients will get 90% better, but may take months
- Patients who are completely paralyzed have been known to regain most of their motor function, even after 1 y to 18 mo of rehabilitation
- Hyponatremia, SVT or heart block, and the usual complications of inactivity (e.g., DVT, pneumonia) are the main complications
- 5% of patients remain permanently disabled
- Vital capacity and negative inspiratory force must be checked frequently for signs of respiratory failure
- 2% recurrence rate

87. Miller-Fisher Syndrome

Etiology/Pathophysiology

- A variant of Guillain-Barré syndrome that presents acutely with a triad of ophthalmoparesis/ptosis, ataxia, and areflexia
- Associated with an antineural antibody (anti-GQ1B)
- Generally occurs following a viral infection
- May present at any age
- Clinical course is similar to GBS

Differential Dx

- GBS
- Myasthenia gravis
- Progressive external ophthalmoplegia
- Lyme disease
- Botulism
- Diphtheria
- Brainstem stroke
- HIV disease
- Tic paralysis
- West Nile virus
- Poliomyelitis

Presentation/Signs & Symptoms

- Similar presentation to GBS
- Generalized weakness
- Flaccidity
- Hypo- or areflexia
- Ataxia of the arms and legs
- Ophthalmoparesis (e.g., ptosis, external ocular muscle weakness) with pupillary sparing
- Dysphagia

Diagnostic Evaluation

- Nerve conduction studies show slowing of nerve conduction velocities, temporal dispersion, conduction block, and absent F waves
- EMG may show irritability and neuropathic potentials, but is not positive for 2 wk
- Serum shows elevated anti-GQ1B antibody
- CSF analysis reveals elevated protein

Treatment/Management

- Recognition of respiratory status is the most important initial management issue
  - Negative inspiratory force and vital capacity can be done at the bedside
  - When vital capacity falls below 15–20 cc/kg (normal 65 cc/kg), V/Q mismatching occurs and intubation may be necessary
- Patients who cannot walk or have abnormal respiratory parameters require inpatient care in a monitored setting; should be treated with IVIG or plasmapheresis ; administer IVIG/plasmapheresis over 5 d within 2 wk of symptom onset
- Anticoagulation for DVT prophylaxis
- Frequent BP checks are necessary as myelinated segments of autonomic nerves can be affected causing rapid swings in BP with increased mortality
- Speech therapy for management of dysphagia

Prognosis/Complications

- Prognosis for walking at 6 mo or improving at least one grade on the MRC scale is dramatically improved in patients receiving IVIG or plasma exchange
- 90% of patients will get 90% better, but may take months
- Patients who are completely paralyzed have been known to regain most of their motor function, even after 1 y to 18 mo of rehabilitation
- Hyponatremia, SVT or heart block, and the usual complications of inactivity (e.g., DVT, pneumonia) are the main complications
- 5% of patients remain permanently disabled
- Vital capacity and negative inspiratory force must be checked frequently for signs of respiratory failure
- 2% recurrence rate

88. Diabetic Neuropathy

Etiology/Pathophysiology

- The most common cause of neuropathy
- 50% of diabetics have some form of neuropathy (entrapment, symmetrical)
- Pathogenesis is controversial
  - Sorbitol theory: Shunting of excess intracellular glucose causes glycosylation of intracellular and extracellular proteins and increased synthesis of fibronectin with proliferation of vascular smooth muscle cells; results in microvessel ischemia in the vasa nervorum
  - Large vessel disease: Arterial disease induced by hyperglycemia chronically results in skin and soft tissue changes and small fiber nerve damage, and distal symmetrical sensory neuropathy
  - Microvascular ischemia: Pure atheromatous disease in microvasculature (brain, retina, and heart) results in chronic ischemia to nerves with resulting mononeuropathy multiplex
- Sensorimotor neuropathies most common; begin in feet; may affect cranial nerves (e.g., cranial nerve III paresis with pupillary sparing, CN VI palsy)
- Autonomic neuropathy is common (e.g., gastroparesis, postural hypotension, impotence)
- Individual nerve involvement may occur (e.g., mononeuritis multiplex, femoral neuropathy, entrapment neuropathy as in carpal tunnel syndrome)

Differential Dx

- Sensorimotor neuropathy
- Uremic neuropathy
- Alcoholic neuropathy
- Vitamin B_6 toxicity
- Vitamin B_{12} deficiency
- Paraneoplastic neuropathy with or without MGUS
- Chronic inflammatory demyelinating polyneuropathy
- Other vitamin deficiency states

Presentation/Signs & Symptoms

- The most common symptom is numbing or burning sensation in the feet with loss of ankle reflexes, followed by involvement of the hands
- Gait disturbance due to loss of position sense in feet
- Loss of vibratory sensation in feet
- Trophic changes in feet (shiny skin)
- Cranial neuropathies, including CN III (pupil usually spared) and VI
- Symptoms of autonomic neuropathies include diarrhea, impotence, postural hypotension, urinary retention
- Mononeuritis multiplex involves large nerves and extremities
- Femoral neuropathy: Pain in top of thigh, weakness of the psoas and quadriceps, loss of knee reflex

Diagnostic Evaluation

- History and physical examination are often diagnostic
- Fasting blood sugar and 2-h glucose tolerance testing are of similar sensitivity in diagnosing diabetes
- Hemoglobin A_{1c} testing has poor screening value but can denote poor sugar control once the diagnosis of diabetes is established
- EMG/nerve conduction studies reveal large fiber (vibratory/proprioception) neuropathy, but is poorly sensitive for small fiber neuropathy
- CSF protein may be elevated

Treatment/Management

- Normalization of fasting sugar to below 110 mg/dL or hemoglobin A_{1c} to less than 7.0
- Physiatry consultation for the appropriate footwear is necessary to decrease the risk of ulceration and eventual amputation and cellulitis
- Desipramine, gabapentin, and phenytoin decrease pain perception by unknown mechanisms
- Duloxepine has recently been approved for pain control
- Entrapment neuropathy may require surgical intervention (e.g., ulnar transposition, carpal tunnel release)
- Postural hypotension is treated with volume expansion, use of TED stockings, Florinef, and α-agonists (e.g., midodrine)
- Other diabetic neuropathies remit with time, such as isolated CN III, IV, and VI neuropathy
- Autonomic neuropathy is disabling and portends high mortality (>30% over 12 mo)

Prognosis/Complications

- The DCCT suggested that normalization of serum glucose can delay initial appearance or progression of peripheral neuropathy
- Autonomic neuropathy in the form of gastroparesis, intractable diarrhea, severe orthostatic hypotension, and intestinal obstruction generally portends poor short-term prognosis
- Cellulitis and amputation are directly related to poor serum glucose control over years
- Isolated sensory peripheral neuropathy has the best chance of improving with excellent sugar control by diet, oral agents, and/or insulin
- The presence of other end organ damage (e.g., retinopathy, stroke, MI, or renal disease with proteinuria) increases the risk that neuropathy is present (>50%)

89. Isolated Sensory Neuropathy

Etiology/Pathophysiology

- A fairly common disorder characterized by a dysesthetic, burning sensation in feet and hands and may include loss of position and vibratory senses
- Most commonly idiopathic, especially in the elderly
- Some etiologies include paraneoplastic syndromes (anti-Hu syndrome), drug toxicities (e.g., Cis-platinum, paclitaxel), acute pyridoxin (vitamin B_6) toxicity, Sjögren's syndrome, HIV disease, and vitamin E deficiency
- Alcoholic neuropathy may present as a predominantly sensory syndrome

Differential Dx

- Sensorimotor neuropathies (e.g., diabetic neuropathy, alcoholic neuropathy)
- Acute myelopathy
- Peripheral vascular disease
- Arsenic intoxication
- Sensory neuropathy associated with cancer

Presentation/Signs & Symptoms

- Numbness and paresthesias in distal extremities
- Dysesthesias (burning pain)
- Gait unsteadiness (sensory ataxia); worse in the dark
- Romberg test present
- Weakness is not present
- Depending on the etiology, presentation may be acute, subacute, or chronic

Diagnostic Evaluation

- History and physical examination, including review of medications and vitamin intake
- Nerve conduction studies reveal absent SNAP
- Check blood for anti-Hu antibodies, ESR, SS-A, SS-B, and HIV testing
- Schirmer test and salivary gland biopsy may be needed to diagnose Sjögren's syndrome
- Screen for underlying malignancy if patient has anti-Hu syndrome

Treatment/Management

- Treat underlying etiology
- Desipramine, gabapentin, and phenytoin decrease pain perception by unknown mechanisms
- Capsaicin cream may provide pain relief

Prognosis/Complications

- Prognosis varies with etiology
- In most cases, successful treatment of the underlying etiology improves the neuropathy (e.g., cessation of offending medication, treatment of vitamin toxicities, treatment of underlying tumors)

90. Entrapment Neuropathy

Etiology/Pathophysiology

- An extremely common type of neuropathy
- A form of traumatic neuropathy
- Various nerves are vulnerable to chronic trauma secondary to passing through narrow, bony, or ligamentous canals
- Pathophysiology generally involves ischemia to the vasa nervorum, resulting in subacute or chronic pathologic changes in myelin and/or axons
- Most commonly involved nerves are the median nerve at the carpal tunnel, ulnar nerve and the cubital tunnel, common peroneal nerve at the fibular head, and radial nerve at the spiral groove of the humerus
- Less commonly involved nerves include the posterior tibial nerve at the tarsal tunnel and the posterior interosseous nerve at the arcade of Frosche
- Activities that compress the nerve will exacerbate symptoms (e.g., typing, knitting, sleeping, and driving for carpal tunnel syndrome; elbow pressure for ulnar neuropathy; squatting or lithotomy position for peroneal neuropathy; sleeping with upper arm in a compressed position for radial neuropathy)

Differential Dx

- Stroke
- Generalized neuropathy
- Mononeuropathy multiplex
- Compartment syndrome
- Peripheral arterial or venous embolization
- Reflex sympathetic dystrophy
- Radiculopathy
- Myelopathy

Presentation/Signs & Symptoms

- Sensory symptoms include tingling (paresthesias) in the distribution of the sensory nerve branches of a single named nerve, numbness, and a "dead" feeling
- Motor symptoms include weakness in the distribution of the motor portion of entrapped nerve
- Skin discoloration
- Hyperalgesia (increased sensitivity to painful stimulus)
- Hyper- or hypoesthesia (increased or decreased sensitivity to touch)
- Tinel's sign (tapping the nerve over the affected area produces paresthesias in its distribution)

Diagnostic Evaluation

- History and physical examination
- EMG and nerve conduction studies identify the site of entrapment
- Imaging to rule out occult fractures and MRI may visualize a compressed median nerve in the carpal tunnel
- Phalen's wrist flexion test is fairly diagnostic for carpal tunnel syndrome

Treatment/Management

- Carpal tunnel syndrome: Splint wrist in neutral position and inject steroid at the carpal tunnel; have patient avoid repetetive tasks
  - Transverse carpal ligament release surgery may be necessary in intractable cases
- Ulnar neuropathy: Avoid leaning on elbows, use soft elbow pad
  - Ulnar nerve transposition surgery may be necessary in intractable cases
- Radial neuropathy: Avoid leaning on arm, splint hand for wrist drop
- Common peroneal neuropathy: Avoid leg crossing, avoid rapid, severe weight loss, use ankle/foot orthosis to avoid Achilles tendon shortening

Prognosis/Complications

- Thyroid disease, DM, cancer, and poor nutrition all produce conditions that predispose to entrapment, as well as generalized neuropathy
- The presence of motor symptoms suggests a worse prognosis than do isolated sensory symptoms
- Splint early when weakness occurs
- EMG/nerve conduction studies can determine whether the process is mostly affecting the myelin or the axon
  - Myelin-predominant entrapments improve with conservative measures
  - Axonal lesions generally portend an incomplete improvement and may suggest the need for surgery to prevent further axon disruption

91. Femoral Neuropathy

Etiology/Pathophysiology

- One of the most common mononeuropathies
- As with other mononeuropathies, etiologies include traumatic, metabolic (e.g., diabetes mellitus), and toxic insults
- Idiopathic disease and diabetic neuropathy are the most common causes
- Pathophysiology involves ischemia to the vasa nervorum, resulting in axonal (more common) and/or demyelinating pathology
- Femoral neuropathy occurring abruptly in a patient on anticoagulation is a neurological emergency and may suggest the presence of a retroperitoneal hemorrhage, especially if coexisting abdominal aortic aneurysm is present

Differential Dx

- L4 radiculopathy
- Anterior lumbar plexopathy
- Hip fracture mimicking femoral innervated muscle weakness
- Retroperitoneal hemorrhage
- Diabetic mononeuropathy
- Compression from a gravid uterus
- Prostate cancer, uterine cancer, or cervical cancer resulting in compression of the lumbar plexus
- Carcinomatous meningitis (cauda equina syndrome)
- Pelvic fracture

Presentation/Signs & Symptoms

- Weakness of knee extension and hip flexion
- Numbness of anterior thigh and medial foreleg
- Lumbar pain with radiation to groin
- Inguinal pain
- Symptoms are usually unilateral; one side may be greatly affected and the other minimally affected
- Decreased or absent patellar jerk

Diagnostic Evaluation

- Detailed neurological history and examination demonstrating knee extension weakness, altered sensation along the anterior thigh and medial foreleg, and lack of weakness of hip adduction and abduction
  - If hip flexion weakness is present, it should be minimal
  - The presence of hip adduction weakness along with knee extension weakness suggests a more proximal lesion of the lumbar plexus or high- and midlumbar roots
- EMG and nerve conduction studies to determine whether symptoms are bilateral in patients with diabetes and to distinguish lumbar radiculopathy and plexopathy from isolated femoral neuropathy
- Lumbar MRI and pelvic imaging to rule out neoplasm or hemorrhage in appropriate patients
- Lumbar puncture if no other cause is found to rule out inflammatory or neoplastic meningeal reaction

Treatment/Management

- Most cases of idiopathic femoral neuropathies improve gradually over the course of 6–18 mo, particularly if blood glucose is controlled
- Physical therapy evaluation, use of a knee stabilizer

Prognosis/Complications

- Patients without neoplastic disease or severe trauma may expect gradual improvement within 6–18 mo
- Faster improvement portends more complete recovery in sensory and motor function
- May rarely worsen over time
- Complications include secondary orthopedic problems (e.g., hip fracture, femoral fracture secondary to falls that result from poor knee stabilization)
- In diabetics, sugar control is of paramount importance
- Can occur in the course of a mononeuropathy multiplex and, therefore, if other mononeuropathies exist, prognosis depends on the medical condition underlying the syndrome

92. Peroneal Neuropathy

Etiology/Pathophysiology

- The most common mononeuropathy of the lower extremity
- Most cases caused by trauma to lateral proximal foreleg where the common peroneal nerve is at its most superficial as it winds around the neck of the fibula
- As in other mononeuropathies, ischemia to the vasa nervorum may cause a "stroke" in the nerve
- Other causes include bleeding near the fibular neck, compressive casts, hyperflexion of the knee in the dorsal lithotomy position during surgical procedures, direct injection of the nerve, and rapid weight loss
- Peroneal neuropathy may occur anywhere on peroneal nerve from lower lumbar plexus to hip area to fibular neck where it ends its course as the common peroneal nerve and branches into deep and superficial branches
- Deep peroneal neuropathy in the anterior compartment of the foreleg may occur with compartment syndrome due to bleeding, swelling, or trauma, resulting in subsequent motor and sensory disability
- Superficial peroneal neuropathy may cause sensory loss along the lateral foreleg and weakness of the lateral compartment muscles
- Many cases of "sciatica" are really misdiagnosed cases of proximal peroneal neuropathy

Differential Dx

- L5 radiculopathy
- Sciatic neuropathy
- Malingering
- Stroke
- Brain or spinal cord tumor compressing foot fibers
- Multiple sclerosis
- Amyotrophic lateral sclerosis
- Contracture
- Peripheral neuropathy
- Charcot-Marie-Tooth syndrome

Presentation/Signs & Symptoms

- Common peroneal nerve: If damaged proximal to the popliteal fossa, mild knee flexion weakness is present with poor foot dorsiflexion, and eversion with preserved inversion
- Common peroneal neuropathy of fibular head (most common): Foot dorsiflexion and eversion weakness occur (resulting in a "steppage" gait); sensory loss along the lateral foreleg and dorsum of foot
- Deep peroneal neuropathy: Foot dorsiflexion weakness, toe extension weakness, and poor sensation in web space on dorsum of foot between first and second toes
- Superficial peroneal neuropathy: Sensory loss of lateral foreleg and dorsum of foot

Diagnostic Evaluation

- History and neurological examination suggests the location of the lesion
  - Almost all cases include some degree of sensory loss
  - If sensory loss does not occur, a careful evaluation is necessary to rule out a motor neuropathy, ALS, or pure motor stroke
  - Patellar and Achilles tendon reflexes are preserved in peroneal neuropathy
  - Peroneal neuropathy is distinguished from L5 radiculopathy by lack of plantar flexion and inversion weakness and sensory loss along the L5 distribution
- Further testing with EMG/nerve conduction studies will further localize the lesion to the fibular head, just proximal to that area, to the hip, or near the piriformis muscle
- Imaging is rarely necessary in peroneal neuropathy (unless the lesion appears to be at the hip) to rule out neoplastic or other compressive causes

Treatment/Management

- Gait training along with ankle/foot orthoses
  - Ankle/foot orthoses to keep the foot from hyperplantar flexion is the best management to prevent Achilles tendon shortening and resultant contracture, which requires corrective surgery
  - Constant care of the ankle/foot orthosis with attention to its proper fitting will help reduce the chance of decubitus and pressure sores
- Pain is rarely a chronic symptom of peroneal neuropathy; thus, analgesics are generally not necessary
- Proximal peroneal neuropathies at the hip or deep in the buttock may require specialized therapy to allow hip stabilization

Prognosis/Complications

- Prognosis depends on the underlying disease
- Generalized processes (e.g., uremia, diabetes) tend to have worse prognoses than isolated traumatic peroneal neuropathy
  - EMG/nerve conduction testing can help determine whether mild or severe neuropathy is occurring and allow accurate prognostication
- Pressure sores from orthoses are common
- Peroneal neuropathy increases the risk for falls due to an increased chance of tripping
- A high index of suspicion for other mononeuropathies is necessary to rule out a more generalized neurogenic disorder

93. Radial Palsy

Etiology/Pathophysiology

- Also referred to as "Saturday Night" palsy
- A compression neuropathy of radial nerve at the spiral groove in the humerus
- Typically occurs when patient gets intoxicated and falls asleep with the arm hanging over a couch or chair
- Most lesions are demyelinating; however, with prolonged compression, axonal loss may occur

Differential Dx

- Other causes of wrist drop
  - C7 radiculopathy
  - Brachial plexus lesion
  - Posterior interosseous neuropathy
  - CNS lesions

Presentation/Signs & Symptoms

- Presents with wrist and finger drop (weakness of wrist and finger extensors)
- Triceps muscles are spared (no weakness of extension at the elbow)
- There is loss of sensation over the lateral dorsal aspect of the hand and first four fingers (in the distribution of superficial radial sensory nerve)

Diagnostic Evaluation

- Nerve conduction studies and EMG help to localize the lesion
- X-ray of the humerus may reveal a fracture
- Cervical MRI if C7 radiculopathy is suspected

Treatment/Management

- Conservative treatment (e.g., wrist and finger splints, physical therapy) is usually adequate, as most cases are self-limited and resolve gradually over time

Prognosis/Complications

- Patients with demyelinating lesions usually recover within weeks
- When lesion is predominantly axonal, recovery may be delayed by months to over a year

94. Alcoholic Neuropathy

Etiology/Pathophysiology

- The second most common cause of peripheral neuropathy in the U.S.; only diabetic neuropathy is more prevalent
- Affects those who drink large quantities of alcohol for many years
  - Many people drink large quantities of alcohol for many years and eat a varied diet and never suffer the disease
  - No precise amount of alcohol intake over a period of time is predictive of alcoholic neuropathy; much depends upon the patient's remaining dietary intake of B vitamins and calories
  - As few as three mixed drinks a day with poor nutritional status can result in the many neurological stigmata of alcoholism
  - Can improve with abstention from alcohol
- The neuropathy is a combined effect of alcohol toxicity and dietary insufficiency, likely of B vitamins
- Pathophysiology involves reduced numbers of large and small myelinated fibers along with axonal degeneration
- Demyelination is not a prominent feature of alcoholic neuropathy

Differential Dx

- Thiamine deficiency
- Diabetes
- Vitamin B_{12} deficiency
- Hypothyroidism
- Paraneoplastic neuropathy
- Restless leg syndrome
- Toxic neuropathy secondary to medications (e.g., metronidazole, chemotherapeutic agents)
- HIV neuropathy

Presentation/Signs & Symptoms

- Loss of position sense causing loss of balance may result in falls and fractures
- Romberg sign reveals balance disparity, with swaying when visual cue removed
- Symmetrical foot numbness
- Foot paresthesias
- May occur subclinically, along with alcoholic dementia
- Patients with alcoholic dementia may have reduced ankle jerks and poor position sense, but do not report the latter symptoms
- Generally does not cause pressure sores as in diabetic neuropathy
- Other stigmata of alcoholism (e.g., liver disease, varices) may occur concurrently

Diagnostic Evaluation

- History and neurologic examination
  - Tests of position sense, vibratory sense, and reflexes will generally reveal hypo- or areflexia distally and poor vibratory sense prior to any symptoms
  - Complete symmetrical anesthesia of the feet and hands generally does not occur as in diabetic and other neuropathies
  - Dementia, history of alcoholism, history of head injury, and seizures may be noted
- CBC may reveal elevated mean corpuscular red cell volume; LFTs may be elevated
- EMG/nerve conduction studies can reveal absent or low-amplitude sensory nerve action potentials with preserved motor responses (motor responses are affected later in the disease process)

Treatment/Management

- Cessation of alcohol intake
- Replete B vitamins, especially vitamin B_{12} and thiamine
- Additional supplementation with folic acid
- Adequate caloric intake
- Physical therapy as necessary to prevent falls
- Home care evaluation may be done to alter the home environment to prevent falls
- Use of a night-light for visual cues when moving around in darker places dramatically decreases the incidence of falls

Prognosis/Complications

- If only sensory symptoms are occurring, prognosis is excellent for recovery, assuming nutritional support and cessation of alcohol intake
- Falls and resultant trauma are the primary complications
- Alcoholic neuropathy is a marker for alcoholic damage to the CNS and the GI tract, and necessitates a workup for occult liver disease and dementia
- Rehabilitation is necessary, as well as psychological support, to prevent a return to heavy alcohol ingestion

95. Heavy Metal Neuropathy

Etiology/Pathophysiology

- Occurs sporadically; usually due to accidental exposure in industrial settings or to environmental contamination
- On occasion, may be due to intentional exposure (e.g., suicide or homicide attempt)
- Common offending agents include mercury, thallium, arsenic, and lead

Differential Dx

- Lead toxicity may have a similar presentation to porphyria
- Arsenic and mercury toxicity may present acutely and be confused with Guillain-Barré syndrome
- Arsenic toxicity may be confused with alcoholic neuropathy or sensory neuropathies

Presentation/Signs & Symptoms

- Mercury toxicity: Paresthesias due to sensory neuropathy, GI symptoms, fatigue, weight loss, tremor, and personality change
- Thallium toxicity: Painful peripheral neuropathy, alopecia, hyperkeratosis, Mees lines on nails, chorea, and ataxia
- Arsenic toxicity similar to thallium toxicity; may also cause a painful peripheral neuropathy with distal weakness, alopecia, Mees lines, GI symptoms (e.g., nausea/vomiting), intracerebral hemorrhage, hyperkeratosis
- Lead in adults mainly a motor neuropathy; may manifest as wrist drop; patients also have associated abdominal colic, anemia, gum discoloring

Diagnostic Evaluation

- Levels of toxins can be measured in urine, blood, nails, and hair
- Nerve conduction studies and EMG help to characterize neuropathy
- Head CT may be useful to evaluate for hemorrhagic encephalopathy in cases of arsenic poisoning

Treatment/Management

- Avoidance of exposure
- Chelation therapy with penicillamine or dimercaptopropanol BAL promotes excretion of toxin

Prognosis/Complications

- With prompt treatment prognosis is often good

96. Mononeuropathy Multiplex

Etiology/Pathophysiology

- Mononeuropathy multiplex refers to multiple isolated nerve injuries resulting in asymmetrical somatic symptoms
- Vasculopathy is then the major cause of the mononeuropathy multiplex syndrome
  - Autoimmune syndromes from systemic disease result in lymphocyte and macrophage infiltration in the vaso nervorum, resulting in nerve ischemia and subsequent sensory and motor symptoms, without necessarily producing the symmetrical symptoms seen in generalized peripheral neuropathy
  - Vasculitis, diabetes, and AIDS are the most common underlying etiologies
- Advanced cases result in a coalescence of multiple asymmetrical mononeuropathies, resulting in symmetrical symptoms that may resemble generalized peripheral neuropathies
- Syndromes may be purely sensory, purely motor, or sensorimotor

Differential Dx

- Guillain-Barré syndrome
- Multifocal motor neuropathy
- Toxic neuropathies due to chemotherapy
- Hereditary neuropathy with liability to pressure palsies
- Multiple nerve entrapments
- Peripheral nerve vasculitis (e.g., small vessel polyarteritis nodosa, Churg-Strauss syndrome, rheumatoid arthritis, Wegener's granulomatosis, cryoglobulinemia)

Presentation/Signs & Symptoms

- As in entrapment neuropathy, pure sensory or sensorimotor symptoms in a variety of dermatomal/myotomal distributions are noted asymmetrically
- Pain is highly prevalent due to the ischemic nature of the disease
- Scapular winging, isolated phrenic nerve palsy, and other unusual mononeuropathies may herald onset of mononeuropathy multiplex
- Unlike generalized peripheral neuropathies, symptoms may occur in the arms as prevalently as in the lower extremity nerves
- Dysphagia and shortness of breath may occur in cranial or phrenic nerve involvement

Diagnostic Evaluation

- History and physical examination, including a detailed history of toxic exposures
  - Weakness, hyporeflexia, sensory symptoms and/or signs of multiple dermatomal/myotomal distributions are necessary for the diagnosis
  - Attempt to establish a primary systemic vasculitis, diabetes, or infectious syndrome as the cause of the patient's symptoms
- Laboratory studies may include fasting blood sugar, ANA, rheumatoid factor, SS-A, SS-B, and ESR
- EMG and NCS can determine an axonal or demyelinating process isolated to multiple named nerves
- Fluoroscopy may be indicated to evaluate for isolated phrenic nerve palsy
- Although CSF analysis for increased protein may detect an ongoing inflammatory process, it is nonspecific so rarely helpful

Treatment/Management

- As with entrapment neuropathies, splinting those joints that are subject to severe weakness can prevent contractures
- Analgesics (e.g., gabapentin, amitriptyline, narcotics) may be useful for ischemic pain
- Treatment of the underlying systemic disease is necessary to prevent ongoing nerve destruction, as most cases are axonal and can result in significant disability
- For many vasculitic etiologies, high-dose oral steroid treatment and/or oral or IV cytotoxic therapy with cyclophosphamide is used
- Physical therapy consultation is necessary if gait and manual dexterity are significantly impaired

Prognosis/Complications

- Prognosis depends upon the underlying systemic disease
- In early diabetes, correction of blood sugar may alleviate the syndrome
- Treatment of rheumatoid arthritis helps its associated mononeuropathy multiplex
- Neoplastic nerve infiltration bodes a poor prognosis

97. Chronic Immune Demyelinating Polyneuropathy

Etiology/Pathophysiology

- CIDP is an autoimmune disorder with similar pathophysiology and presentation as Guillain-Barré syndrome, but has a chronic course
- Cell mediated and humoral responses against myelin have been demonstrated
- Onset or relapses may be triggered by infections or immunizations
- Usually afflicts patients between 30 and 50 years of age
- Disease is slightly more common in men
- Has a prolonged course marked by relapses and remissions

Differential Dx

- Other causes of peripheral neuropathy
  - GBS
  - Diabetic polyneuropathy
  - Heavy metal poisoning
  - Vasculitic neuropathy
  - Nutritional neuropathy

Presentation/Signs & Symptoms

- Weakness
  - Usually symmetrical
  - Affects both proximal and distal muscles
- Absent or diminished deep tendon reflexes are a hallmark of the disease
- Sensory deficits occur frequently
- Cranial nerve involvement (e.g., facial and bulbar weakness, ophthalmoparesis) may be seen on rare occasions

Diagnostic Evaluation

- Nerve conduction studies show slowing of conduction velocities, conduction blocks, dispersion of responses, and prolonged distal latencies
- CSF analysis reveals elevated protein with few cells
- Sural nerve biopsy shows demyelination, at times with onion bulb formation and endoneural inflammatory infiltrates

Treatment/Management

- Responds well to immunomodulating therapy: Corticosteroids, IVIG, plasmapheresis, azathioprine, and cyclophosphamide all have been shown to be effective
- In some refractory patients, combination therapy may work better

Prognosis/Complications

- Majority of patients respond favorably to immunomodulating therapy
- Full recovery in 80% of cases

98. Myasthenia Gravis

Etiology/Pathophysiology

- An autoimmune disease caused by the development of antibodies to acetylcholine receptors at the neuromuscular junction, which inhibit muscle membrane depolarization
- Results in interference of neuromuscular transmission leading to muscular weakness
- Pathogenesis may begin in the thymic tissue, which provides an area for autoantibody production in susceptible patients
- There is a 20% concurrence with autoimmune hypothyroidism, suggesting a more generalized autoimmune disorder
- Associated with thymic hyperplasia in 80% of cases, thymoma in 15% of cases (30% of these are malignant), thyrotoxicosis, rheumatoid arthritis, SLE
- Occurs primarily in young women and older men; may occur at any age
- Myasthenic crises are associated with infections and may result in respiratory muscle weakness necessitating intubation
- Congenital myasthenia is rare and is relatively refractory to treatment
- Neonatal myasthenia occurs in 12% of pregnancies to myasthenic women via placental transfer of anti-acetylcholine receptor antibodies

Differential Dx

- Guillain-Barré syndrome
- Botulism
- Lambert-Eaton syndrome
- Nondepolarizing muscle relaxants
- Brainstem stroke
- Ocular myopathy
- Thyroid disease
- Cranial neuropathy
- Tic paralysis
- Organophosphate poisoning
- ALS
- D-Penicillamine (temporary reaction)

Presentation/Signs & Symptoms

- Fatigable weakness
  - Ocular and facial muscles are most frequently involved (diplopia, ptosis, dysphagia, drooling, difficulty chewing); 75% of cases are restricted to ocular involvement
  - Symmetrical limb weakness
  - Respiratory failure due to respiratory muscle weakness
  - Weakness often fluctuates
  - Especially prominent following persistent activity
- Head lolling (inability to hold up head)
- Symptoms may be subtle as to suggest hysteria
- Normal reflexes, cerebellar, and sensory function

Diagnostic Evaluation

- Subacute onset of fluctuating diplopia and ptosis with normal pupillary responses strongly suggests myasthenia gravis
- Anticholinergic challenge with edrophonium will rapidly and temporarily reverse symptoms in most patients
  - Used for the initial diagnosis
  - Also used to distinguish myasthenic crisis (worsening of disease) versus cholinergic crisis (supratherapeutic drug levels secondary to medications): Edrophonium will reverse myasthenic crisis but exacerbate cholinergic crisis
- Acetylcholine receptor antibody assay positive in >80%
- Routine laboratory tests and CSF is normal
- TSH is often abnormal
- Imaging of mediastinum to rule out thymoma
- Repetitive nerve stimulation results in a decremental response in motor unit amplitude
- Single-fiber EMG is the most sensitive test

Treatment/Management

- Symptomatic treatment with acetylcholinesterase inhibitors (e.g., neostigmine, pyridostigmine) allows more time for acetylcholine to compete for binding and active acetylcholine receptor sites, thereby allowing the patient to maintain strength
- Frequent measurement of vital capacity and negative inspiratory force is necessary to evaluate respiratory muscle function; intubation may be necessary
- Corticosteroids (must start slowly as high initial doses may worsen the disease), IVIG, and immunosuppressive agents (e.g., azathioprine, cyclosporine, methotrexate, mycophenolate)
- Plasmapheresis for severe cases, myasthenic crises
- Thymectomy may be curative; cure may take months
- Avoid immunoglycosides, sedative hypnotics, β-blockers, and other medications that may decrease neuromuscular transmission

Prognosis/Complications

- If disease is diagnosed early and appropriate supportive measures are taken, mortality is low
- Characterized by remissions and exacerbations of fluctuating weakness, but does not follow a steadily progressive course
- If limited to ocular muscles for >2 y, it rarely extends to other muscles
- Patients with a forced vital capacity <1.5 liters usually require prophylactic intubation or at least observation in an ICU
- Patients should be admitted if they cannot walk or have signs of respiratory distress
- Starting steroids without the direction of a neurological consultant is discouraged

99. Botulism

Etiology/Pathophysiology

- Botulism is caused by *Clostridium botulinum*, a gram-positive, anaerobic, spore-forming bacillus that produces neurotoxins that irreversibly bind to neuromuscular junctions
- Botulinum toxin poisoning is a presynaptic disease: Release of acetylcholine is inhibited at the neuromuscular junction, thereby interfering with transmission of nerve impulses and resulting in weakness and paralysis
- There are three clinical syndromes caused by botulism
  - Foodborne botulism: Typically follows ingestion of canned food or contaminated seafood that contain the preformed toxin
  - Infant botulism: Currently the most common worldwide cause; occurs due to colonization of infant gut by toxin-producing bacteria
  - Wound botulism: Due to colonization and toxin production in traumatized tissues; seen in IV drug abusers with abscesses
- Incubation time 12–36 h (infant botulism 3–30 d)

Differential Dx

- Myasthenia gravis
- Guillain-Barré syndrome
- Lambert-Eaton syndrome
- Sepsis
- Anticholinergic poisoning
- Poliomyelitis
- Intoxications (e.g., cocaine)
- Tetanus

Presentation/Signs & Symptoms

- The syndrome frequently begins with gastroenteritis
- Sudden onset of descending paralysis
  - Usually occurs 12–72 h following ingestion of toxin
  - Symmetrical, flaccid paralysis
- Diplopia, ptosis, dysphagia, and dysarthria (presents as nasal speech) occur early
- Blurring of vision occurs due to paralysis of accommodation
- Dysautonomia manifesting as dryness of mouth, paralytic ileus, urinary retention
- Weakness of respiratory muscles may lead to acute respiratory failure

Diagnostic Evaluation

- Serum, stool, or wound can be tested for toxin
- Stool should be cultured for *C. botulinum*
- Contaminated food should be tested for both toxin and organism
- Rapid nerve stimulation studies reveal incremental responses typical of presynaptic disease

Treatment/Management

- Early administration of human-derived trivalent antitoxin should be administered as early as possible
- Guanidine and 4-aminopyridine have been reported to improve weakness in some patients
- Vitals should be monitored closely in an ICU setting
- Patients often require ventilatory support
- Secondary infections may occur; however, antibiotics are generally avoided because they may increase toxin release and worsen clinical status
- Do not use aminoglycosides, as they contribute to neuromuscular blockade and worsen the patient's condition

Prognosis/Complications

- Complete recovery can be expected with optimal treatment, though improvement may take weeks to months
- Mortality may be as low as 1% or as high as 50%, depending on severity of illness and adequacy of treatment
- Recovery takes up to several weeks, even with ideal treatment
- 75% of patients with botulism have respiratory failure requiring intubation; if treated before hypoxic episodes occur, full recovery is likely
- Recovery from foodborne disease does not result in immunity to botulinum toxin

100. Lambert-Eaton Myasthenic Syndrome

Etiology/Pathophysiology

- Also referred to as "myasthenic syndrome"
- A presynaptic neuromuscular disease often associated with small-cell lung carcinoma, which produces an antibody to voltage-gated calcium channels preventing calcium accumulation within the nerve terminal, which are necessary for presynaptic release of acetylcholine and subsequent muscle contraction
  - Association with malignancy or autoimmune disease in >80% of cases
  - More than 80% of the malignancies associated with LES are small-cell carcinoma of the lung
  - Can occur in association with rectal carcinoma, renal carcinoma, basal cell carcinoma, and lymphoreticular malignancies
- Affects men twice as commonly as women
- The syndrome can occur before the clinical onset of the associated autoimmune or neoplastic disease
- Similar to "stiff person syndrome"; antibodies are also produced as a paraneoplastic or autoimmune phenomenon, although target epitope differs
- Any significant weakness that occurs in a patient with small-cell carcinoma of the lung should necessitate a specific workup for LES

Differential Dx

- Polymyositis
- Dermatomyositis
- Myasthenia gravis
- Inclusion body myopathy
- Late-onset muscular dystrophies
- Proximal myotonic dystrophy
- Cervical spinal cord compression
- Amyotrophic lateral sclerosis
- Stiff person syndrome
- Hysteria/malingering

Presentation/Signs & Symptoms

- Proximal upper- and lower-extremity weakness and myalgias
  - Improves with activity (unlike myasthenia gravis)
  - May be mistaken for weakness and fatigue due to chemotherapy and cancer
  - Weakness precedes identification of the underlying autoimmune or neoplastic disease in many cases and should necessitate a workup for lung neoplasia
- Reflexes more active after than before exercise
- May cause dry mouth or constipation, but extraocular muscles are spared (unlike myasthenia gravis)
- May cause dysphagia and neck weakness

Diagnostic Evaluation

- EMG and NCS reveal normal sensory potentials and very low amplitude motor potentials, mimicking a myopathy or motor neuron disease
  - Repetitive stimulation of motor nerves at 2–3 Hz will show a decrement in amplitude, as in myasthenia gravis
  - Repetitive stimulation after exercise or with a 50-Hz train of stimulation results in a dramatic increase in motor unit action potential amplitude; an increase of >100% is diagnostic of a presynaptic disorder (e.g., LES, botulism)
- The ultimately specific test is demonstration of elevated titers of voltage gated calcium channel antibodies
- If LES is established in a patient without other significant medical disease, then a serious workup should be performed to rule out occult neoplasia, including chest CT and bronchoscopy
- Test for ANA, SS-A, SS-B, ESR, and rheumatoid factor

Treatment/Management

- Supportive care is the mainstay of treatment, including intubation if necessary, treatment of pressure sores, DVT prophylaxis
- Immunomodulating agents, such as prednisone, IVIG, and plasmapheresis, all improve the syndrome by removing the offending antibody or altering its production
- Specific attempts to increase acetylcholine vesicle release with guanidine and 4-aminopyridine are also useful
  - 4-aminopyridine is preferred to guanidine but may cause seizures
- Successful treatment of the underlying neoplasm may improve LES in some cases
- Use of pyridostigmine may help minimally

Prognosis/Complications

- Prognosis depends upon the mortality and morbidity of the underlying disease
- Therefore, treatment of LES is frequently a quality-of-life issue rather than an improvement-in-mortality issue
- Those patients with idiopathic or autoimmune-related disease generally suffer increased morbidity and mortality
- This disease is underdiagnosed and should be part of the workup for any individual with occult weakness without sensory loss

101. Inclusion Body Myositis

Etiology/Pathophysiology

- A common form of myopathy that affects the distal muscles as much as proximal muscles, unlike other myopathies
- The most common inflammatory myopathy in adults
- Previously diagnosed as "steroid-unresponsive polymyositis"
- Controversy exists as to whether this is a primary degenerative muscle disease, as amyloid has been noted in specimens, or whether this is a primary immune-mediated disease as indicated by the inflammatory pathology
  - Pathology is similar to polymyositis; however, electron microscopy reveals inclusion bodies in the muscle (e.g., rimmed vacuoles, cytoplasmic whorls)
  - Evidence that this is a degenerative disease comes from failure of trials of anti-inflammatory medications
  - Lymphocytic infiltration, variation in fiber size, presence of regenerating fibers, and an increase in interstitial tissue all suggest an immune-mediated syndrome
- Sporadic and familial varieties exist
- Affects males more commonly than females

Differential Dx

- Polymyositis
- Dermatomyositis
- Amyotrophic lateral sclerosis
- Lambert-Eaton syndrome
- Adult onset inherited myopathies
- Myasthenia gravis
- Cervical spinal cord disease
- Oculopharyngeal muscular dystrophy

Presentation/Signs & Symptoms

- Insidious onset of proximal upper and lower extremity weakness in patients age >50 y, particularly men
  - Quadriceps and finger flexor weakness are most common, along with dysphagia; however, any pattern of symmetrical muscle weakness may occur
- Dysphagia is very common
- Significant muscle atrophy may occur, along with hypo- or areflexia
- The course does not fluctuate as in myasthenia gravis
- Sensory loss, cramps, and fasciculations are absent
- Ptosis and diplopia do not occur
- Bowel and bladder are not affected

Diagnostic Evaluation

- Workup is similar for all pure motor weakness syndromes without sensory loss (e.g., inclusion body myositis, ALS, myasthenia gravis)
- Laboratory studies include ESR (normal) and CK (may be elevated in 50% of cases, depending on the rapidity of muscle degeneration)
- EMG and nerve conduction studies show a bizarre combination of myopathic and neurogenic features due to muscle destruction by terminal axonal damage
- Muscle biopsy is diagnostic, revealing lymphocytic infiltration, variation in muscle fiber size, evidence of regenerating fibers, and presence of vacuoles and cytoplasmic whorls via electron microscopy

Treatment/Management

- Immunomodulating agents have not been shown to be beneficial
- Steroids do not alter the clinical course
- Physiatry consultation for bracing and exercises
- It is imperative to make the correct diagnosis to rule out treatable myopathies (e.g., polymyositis, dermatomyositis)
- Dysphagia suggests a poor clinical course and percutaneous gastrostomy may be necessary

Prognosis/Complications

- Most patients become significantly disabled within 10 y, either becoming wheelchair-bound or requiring alternative methods of feeding
- Clinical course is not as severe as that of ALS
- The usual complications of immobility are common, including decubitus ulcers, DVT, pneumonia from aspiration, and chronic pain from joint contractures
- Further studies evaluating a potential link between this disease and Alzheimer-type dementia due to the presence of amyloid may be fruitful

102. Duchenne Muscular Dystrophy

Etiology/Pathophysiology

- The most common and deadly form of muscular dystrophy
- An X-linked recessive disorder resulting in deletions, duplications, and point mutations in the dystrophin gene
- The dystrophin protein normally acts between subsarcolemmal proteins to anchor the sarcomeres through extracellular structural proteins allowing normal muscle integrity
- In Duchenne muscular dystrophy, there is an absence of dystrophin, causing aberrant muscle maturation and subsequent degeneration and resultant muscle weakness
- Some mutations lead to dystrophin fragments produced in less severe disease (e.g., Becker muscular dystrophy in which weakness is mild)
- The discovery of this gene and gene product has made it easier to define other muscular dystrophies and the importance to subsarcolemmal and extracellular proteins in maintaining muscle cell integrity
- Female carriers may be mildly affected

Differential Dx

- Becker muscular dystrophy
- Congenital muscular dystrophy
- Spinomuscular atrophy
- Childhood myasthenia gravis
- Childhood dermatomyositis or polymyositis
- Myotonic dystrophy
- Chronic inflammatory demyelinating polyneuropathy
- Emery-Dreifuss muscular dystrophy

Presentation/Signs & Symptoms

- Affected patients are healthy males at birth
- Mildly delayed motor milestones occur
- Clumsy, waddling gait; slow running; difficulty rising from seated position and climbing stairs begins around ages 4–5
- Enlarged calves due to perimysial scarring may be incongruously evident
- Pelvic and shoulder girdle weakness with preserved reflexes
- Toe walking is common
- Exaggerated lumbar lordosis
- Gower's sign: Child climbs up from a seated position while holding onto his own limbs
- Bulbar muscles are generally spared

Diagnostic Evaluation

- ECG may reveal prominent R waves in the anterior and septal leads and deep Q waves in the lateral leads
- Extremely elevated CK levels are common
- EMG reveals a myopathic pattern, including short, sharp, abundant potentials
- Muscle biopsy reveals dystrophic changes, including perimysial scarring, variation in fiber size, lymphocytic infiltration, and futile attempts at muscle cell regeneration
- Genetic testing for changes in the dystrophin gene or immunocytofluorescence revealing a complete absence of dystrophin in muscle tissue is diagnostic
- Genetic testing differentiates between the fatal muscular dystrophy and nonfatal variants, such as Becker muscular dystrophy, where dystrophin fragments are present
- Previous family history of weakness in an X-linked recessive pattern may be helpful

Treatment/Management

- Treatment is primarily supportive
- Prevention of contractures with active and passive stretching
- Extended life is possible with respiratory support
- Prednisone may stabilize strength briefly but does not change the inevitable terminal course of the disease
- Attempts at gene transfer techniques have failed to produce dystrophin; however, further attempts at gene therapy and insertion are still being studied

Prognosis/Complications

- Death occurs by the third to early fourth decades of life
- Mortality usually occurs due to cardiomyopathy and/or respiratory failure
- Longer-lived patients may develop some intellectual decline due to cerebral effects of absent dystrophin

103. Limb-Girdle Muscular Dystrophy

Etiology/Pathophysiology

- Limb-girdle muscular dystrophy applies to a heterogeneous group of syndromes each with a distinct genetic mutation that present with progressive proximal weakness
- Most cases are autosomal-recessive, though some may have an autosomal-dominant pattern of inheritance
- Begins in late childhood or early adolescence
- Subtypes include sarcoglycanopathies, Fukutin-related proteinopathy, calpainopathy, and dysferlinopathy
- Other subtypes extremely rare and reported only in specific pedigrees

Differential Dx

- Other forms of muscular dystrophy (e.g., Duchenne muscular dystrophy, fascioscapulohumeral dystrophy)
- Congenital myopathies
- Metabolic myopathies (e.g., acid maltase myopathy, carnitine deficiency)
- Mitochondrial myopathy
- Thyrotoxic myopathy
- Polymyositis

Presentation/Signs & Symptoms

- The course of illness and pattern of weakness varies with the subtype of disease
- Proximal limb girdle weakness is common to all types
- Facial muscles are spared
- Calf hypertrophy, scoliosis, lordosis, and joint contractures are seen in some subtypes
- Cardiac involvement is absent

Diagnostic Evaluation

- CK levels are elevated variably (mildly in some patients but markedly in others)
- EMG reveals a myopathic pattern of abnormalities, including short, sharp, abundant potentials without denervation
- Muscle biopsy shows dystrophic changes with muscle necrosis
- Muscle immunohistology is helpful in some cases
- Genetic studies may be useful

Treatment/Management

- There is no cure available for these disorders
- Physical therapy and orthotics

Prognosis/Complications

- Prognosis varies depending on the subtype
- Most types have a progressive decline
- Patients often become wheelchair-bound
- Patients usually succumb to pulmonary complications (e.g., pneumonia, pulmonary embolus)

104. Fascioscapulohumeral Muscular Dystrophy

Etiology/Pathophysiology

- A rare muscle disease that leads to atrophy of the shoulder and facial muscles
- Autosomal dominant inheritance pattern that results in a gene defect on chromosome 4q35
- The underlying pathophysiology of muscle degeneration and necrosis is unclear
- The disease manifests in adolescence or adult life

Differential Dx

- Other forms of muscular dystrophy (e.g., limb girdle muscular dystrophy, Emery-Dreifuss dystrophy)
- Inflammatory myopathies
- Mitochondrial myopathies
- Spinomuscular atrophy
- Congenital myopathies (e.g., centronuclear myopathy)
- Metabolic myopathies (e.g., acid maltase deficiency)
- Scapuloperoneal syndrome

Presentation/Signs & Symptoms

- Weakness of shoulder girdle muscles, neck muscles, and facial muscles
  - Asymmetrical weakness is common
  - Winging of scapula is present
  - Biceps and triceps are weak and atrophic, whereas deltoid and forearm muscles are spared
  - Facial muscle weakness signs: Pouting lips, horizontal smile, and inability to whistle or drink through a straw
- Abdominal muscles are usually weak, resulting in a protuberant abdomen and exaggerated lordosis
- In the lower extremities, the dorsiflexors are most involved, causing foot drop
- Cardiac involvement is rare

Diagnostic Evaluation

- Serum CK levels are usually mild to moderately elevated
- EMG reveals nonspecific myopathic changes, but is usually helpful to rule out neuropathic conditions
- Muscle biopsy shows nonspecific myopathic changes and is not useful in establishing the diagnosis
- Diagnosis can be confirmed with DNA analysis

Treatment/Management

- There is no specific treatment for this condition
- Physical therapy

Prognosis/Complications

- Patients have a normal lifespan
- Weakness develops gradually and patients may remain ambulatory well into the fifth or sixth decades of life

105. Congenital Myopathies

Etiology/Pathophysiology

- A group of nonprogressive muscle disorders that result in minimal weakness
- More than several dozen specific types exist (e.g., central core myopathy, nemaline myopathy, centronuclear myopathy, myopathy with tubular aggregates), which are identified by their characteristic histopathology
- May be classified into those types that are purely muscular dystrophies versus those that have cerebral involvement in addition to muscle disease
- These are extremely rare conditions with dominant, recessive, or X-linked inheritance
- Required for the diagnosis is a clinical examination consistent with weakness, the presence of myopathy seen on muscle biopsy, and EMG with myopathic changes near the time of birth
- A variety of causes are being elucidated; most involve synthesis of proteins required to maintain the sarcolemma, including myosin, tropomyosin, merosin, and others
- Usually presents at birth or shortly thereafter; however, may rarely present with gradual onset myopathy in childhood and adulthood

Differential Dx

- Spinomuscular atrophy (Werdnig-Hoffman disease)
- Congenital myotonic dystrophy
- Neonatal systemic disease (e.g., sepsis)
- Congenital brain and spinal cord malformations causing a floppy infant
- Congenital or neonatal myasthenia gravis

Presentation/Signs & Symptoms

- "Floppy infant" (poor muscle tone)
- Respiratory failure near birth
- Poor spontaneous limb movement
- Tachypnea
- Orthopnea
- Hypoxemia
- Failure to reach appropriate motor milestones at 3, 6, and 12 mo
- Skeletal deformities (suggesting weakness in utero)
- Dysmorphic features with intact reflexes

Diagnostic Evaluation

- CK may be normal or mildly elevated
- Brain and spinal cord imaging to rule out congenital central nervous system anomalies
- EMG and nerve conduction studies may reveal a neurogenic or myopathic process
- Muscle biopsy is diagnostic
- Electromicroscopy frequently reveals disruption of the rigid sarcomere structure and disruption of the Z-disc, as well as abnormal accumulations or decreased presence of anchoring proteins allowing sarcomere disruption over time

Treatment/Management

- There are no specific treatments for any of these conditions
- Avoidance of anesthetic agents that may promote malignant hyperthermia
- Immunomodulating agents are not useful
- Genetic counseling is indicated for those conditions with known inheritance
- Attention to respiratory and orthopedic care

Prognosis/Complications

- No reliable prognosis can be given to any particular patient with congenital myopathy
- Some patients die shortly after birth while others survive many years
- Progression of disease in most patients is generally quite slow
- Some patients with nemaline myopathy are diagnosed only as adults
- Disabled patients may suffer from DVT, pneumonia, or cellulitis
- Some myopathies are associated with mental retardation

106. Mitochondrial Myopathies

Etiology/Pathophysiology

- This is a heterogeneous group of disorders with genetic defects in mitochondrial DNA
- The abnormalities in the mitochondria cause impaired ATP synthesis, resulting in weakness and fatigue
- Recent advances in molecular genetics have identified multiple mitochondrial DNA mutations, each leading to a specific syndrome
- The varied and diverse presentations of mitochondrial myopathies pose a challenge to pinpoint the exact syndrome, particularly since some syndromes may have overlapping features
- These syndromes have multisystem involvement
- These syndromes do not follow mendelian inheritance pattern but instead are transmitted exclusively by mother to progeny
- Kearns-Sayre syndrome: Progressive external ophthalmoplegia with systemic disease (e.g., cardiac conduction defects, hearing loss, ataxia)
- Mitochondrial encephalopathy, lactic acidosis and stroke-like episodes (MELAS): Strokes occur at young ages, may develop seizures or dementia
- Myoclonus epilepsy with ragged red fibers (MERRF): A syndrome highlighted by myoclonic epilepsy and ataxia; some may develop dementia

Differential Dx

- Congenital myopathies
- Myasthenia gravis
- Refsum disease
- Myotonic dystrophy
- Zidovudine may lead to myopathy with ragged red fibers

Presentation/Signs & Symptoms

- Common clinical features in all types include ptosis and progressive external ophthalmoparesis, short stature with decreased muscle mass, proximal weakness, poor endurance and early fatigue, and sensorineural hearing loss
- Kearns-Sayre: Pigmentary retinopathy, myopathy, cerebellar ataxia, hearing loss, and cardiac conduction blocks
- MELAS: CVA at young age, seizures, dementia, myopathic weakness, migraine headaches, recurrent nausea/vomiting
- MERRF: Myoclonic epilepsy, ataxia, dementia, exercise intolerance, lactic acidosis

Diagnostic Evaluation

- Resting serum lactate and pyruvate levels are usually elevated
- ECG may show conduction blocks
- CSF studies reveal elevated protein and high lactate and pyruvate levels
- EMG reveals myopathic changes
- Brain imaging studies may show atrophy and basal ganglia calcification
- Muscle biopsy shows ragged red fibers on Gomori trichrome stain, which are the hallmark of mitochondrial myopathy
- Molecular genetics and respiratory chain enzyme assays can be used to confirm diagnosis

Treatment/Management

- There is no specific treatment available
- Antioxidants (e.g., coenzyme Q_{10}, vitamin C, vitamin E, β-carotene) have been recommended
- Seizure prophylaxis
- Antiplatelet medications (e.g., aspirin, clopidogrel) to reduce risk of recurrent stroke

Prognosis/Complications

- Prognosis varies with clinical syndrome
- Patients are usually impaired as a result of strokes, seizures, weakness, hearing loss, and visual disturbances

107. Inflammatory Myopathies

Etiology/Pathophysiology

- These are autoimmune disorders associated with muscle inflammation, leading to muscle necrosis and proximal, bilateral muscle weakness
- Three types are seen in clinical practice: Polymyositis, dermatomyositis, and inclusion body myositis (this entry discusses polymyositis and dermatomyositis)
- The most common acquired causes of muscle weakness
- May be associated with mixed connective tissue diseases and other autoimmune diseases (e.g., scleroderma, rheumatoid arthritis, SLE)
- Some cases are related to systemic cancers
- Females > males (2:1)

Differential Dx

- Muscular dystrophies
- Viral myositis
- Inclusion body myositis
- Thyrotoxic myopathy
- Hypothyroidism
- Cushing's disease
- Myasthenia gravis

Presentation/Signs & Symptoms

- Subacute onset of symmetrical, predominantly proximal weakness
- Myalgias occur in half of patients
- Dermatomyositis has a characteristic heliotropic (purplish) rash that is seen on the upper eyelids and an erythematous rash on the knuckles (Gottron's patches), neck, shoulders, and extensor surfaces
- Systemic symptoms may occur (e.g., fever, fatigue, arthralgias)
- Dysphagia may occur (due to involvement of striated muscle in the upper third of esophagus)

Diagnostic Evaluation

- CK level is markedly elevated (up to 50 times normal)
  - Elevations of CK precede weakness by several weeks
- Other elevated enzymes include aldolase, myoglobin, LDH, glutamate, pyruvate
- ANA may be positive
- Electromyography shows distinct abnormalities in the involved muscles, including a combination of neuropathic and myopathic features
- Muscle biopsy is helpful to confirm the diagnosis
- Dermatomyositis may be diagnosed by the characteristic rash without muscle findings

Treatment/Management

- Treatment is aimed at increasing muscle strength
- Immunosuppressive therapy is used, primarily high-dose corticosteroids
  - Discontinue if strength does not improve in 3 mo (3/4 patients fail to improve with steroids)
- Other agents, such as azathioprine and methotrexate, may be used for patients that cannot tolerate corticosteroids or for steroid sparing
- Some patients respond temporarily to IVIG
- Physical therapy

Prognosis/Complications

- Symptoms progress over weeks to months or even years
- Immunosuppressive therapy is generally effective
- Dermatomyositis has the better prognosis (80% 5-y survival)
- Most deaths occur from pulmonary or cardiac complications, including conduction defects, arrhythmias, dilated cardiomyopathy, interstitial lung disease, and pulmonary dysfunction
- Other complications include joint contractures and subcutaneous calcifications
- Increased incidence of neoplasia, especially breast, ovarian, colon, and melanoma
- Milder disease occurs in patients with coexisting rheumatoid arthritis, SLE, scleroderma, and Sjögren's syndrome

108. Myotonic Dystrophy

Etiology/Pathophysiology

- Myotonic dystrophy is an inherited disorder of muscle and multiple organs
- Due to an autosomal-dominant inheritance pattern with variable penetrance that results in CTG trinucleotide repeats
- Primarily a muscle disease, resulting in weakness, atrophy, and myotonia; however, the condition is systemic and affects the endocrine, cardiac, pulmonary, and GI systems in addition to muscle; cognition may also be impaired
- The most common form of dystrophy in adults
- Usually manifests in the third or fourth decades of life

Differential Dx

- Inflammatory myopathies (e.g., dermatomyositis, polymyositis, inclusion body myositis)
- Muscular dystrophies
- Mitochondrial myopathies
- Channelopathies that present with myotonia (e.g., hyperkalemic periodic paralysis, congenital myotonia)

Presentation/Signs & Symptoms

- Initially presents with weakness of facial, sternocleidomastoid, and distal limb muscles
- Atrophy occurs primarily in the facial and neck musculature
- Myotonia is present in all muscle groups
- Presenile cataracts and ptosis common
- Male balding pattern
- Cardiac conduction blocks are common, which may clinically manifest as syncope
- Endocrine abnormalities may include diabetes mellitus and testicular atrophy
- GI involvement may be present, including dysphagia and pseudointestinal obstruction

Diagnostic Evaluation

- History and physical examination may reveal multiple organ involvement
- EMG reveals the characteristic abnormal high-frequency discharges that wax and wane, sound like a "dive bomber," and are referred to as electrical myotonia; this is a hallmark of all myotonic syndromes
- Muscle biopsy shows muscle fiber necrosis and fibrosis but changes are not pathognomonic for the disease
- CK levels may be mildly elevated
- ECG, testosterone levels, glucose tolerance test, and pulmonary function studies should be done
- Genetic testing for myotonic dystrophy is commercially available

Treatment/Management

- Muscle stiffness due to myotonia can be relieved with phenytoin, mexiletine, procainamide, or quinine
- Regular cardiac evaluation and possible need for pacemaker
  - Patients should be closely monitored with frequent ECGs and Holter monitoring for worsening cardiac conduction blocks
- Braces may improve ambulation

Prognosis/Complications

- Patients may die early form cardiac problems, aspiration pneumonia, or respiratory failure
- Mild to moderate mental retardation occurs with advancement of the disease
- Personality disorders frequently occur
- Life expectancy is reduced

109. Muscle Channelopathies

Etiology/Pathophysiology

- Varied group of disorders of nerve and muscle, caused by disordered axon potential generation or channel blockage secondary to abnormal Na^+, K^+, or Ca^{2+} membrane channels; result in periodic paralysis and/or myotonia
- These are very uncommon conditions that are generally caused by inherited disorders (autosomal-dominant); nerve channelopathies may be caused by toxin ingestion (often from fish)
- Some of these disorders represent autoimmune attacks via antibody or antibody/complement interactions that either destroy them or cause transient abnormal electrical conduction
- Some disorders of muscle/nerve membrane conduction slowing are probably wrongfully attributed to demyelination or muscle destruction, but are actually likely the result of reversible channelopathies
- Chloride channel: Congenital myotonia (Thomsen's disease)
- Sodium channel: Hyperkalemic periodic paralysis, paramyotonia congenita
- Calcium channel: Hypokalemic periodic paralysis
  - Due to failure of repolarization of the sarcoplasmic reticulum, resulting in weakness during periods of mild hypokalemia
  - Attacks are generally precipitated by a high-carbohydrate meal and/or strenuous exercise followed by sleep

Differential Dx

- Peripheral neuropathy
- Myopathy
- Myasthenia gravis
- Botulism
- Lambert-Eaton myasthenic syndrome
- Guillain-Barré syndrome
- Brainstem stroke
- Drug intoxication
- Hysteria
- Myelopathy
- Thyrotoxicosis
- Acute intermittent porphyria
- Cervical spinal cord disease
- Hysteria/malingering

Presentation/Signs & Symptoms

- Channelopathies are associated with periodic weakness and/or myotonia (failure of a contracted muscle to relax)
- May be associated with cramps or myalgias
- Congenital myotonia: Onset in childhood or adolescence; resulting in large muscles that become "frozen" after contraction
- Hyperkalemic paralysis: Myotonia, periodic paralysis associated with mild hyperkalemia
- Hypokalemia paralysis: Reversible attacks of mild to severe weakness associated with mild hypokalemia; myotonia is absent

Diagnostic Evaluation

- History and physical examination: Congenital diseases may be suggested by family history of severe weakness; a history of paralysis following rest after a period of exercise suggests the periodic paralysis disorders; history of fish ingestion
- Laboratory studies include serum electrolytes, CK, thyroid function tests
- EMG and NCS are routinely normal; reveal myotonic discharges in congenital myotonia and hyperkalemic paralysis
- Provocative tests may be used to induce attacks for diagnosis
  - Administration of glucose and insulin will drive potassium into cells, thereby provoking an attack of hypokalemic paralysis
  - Administration of potassium will elevate serum potassium to provoke an attack of hyperkalemic paralysis
- Genetic testing is not commercially available

Treatment/Management

- Treatment is directed at relaxation of muscles and avoidance of vigorous activity
- Congenital myotonia: Quinine, procainamide, and phenytoin may prevent myotonic episodes
- Hyperkalemic periodic paralysis: Responds to acetazolamide and other diuretics; avoid high carbohydrate meals
- Hypokalemic periodic paralysis: Responds to small doses of K^+ and acetazolamide; avoid high-carbohydrate meals; treat associated thyrotoxicosis
  - Administration of oral potassium during attacks lessens the severity of the attack
  - Acetazolamide induces metabolic acidosis, preventing intracellular shift of K^+ and weakness
- Counseling to prevent frequency and severity of attacks will decrease risk of fixed muscle weakness over time

Prognosis/Complications

- Untreated, repeated attacks can lead to permanent weakness
- Attacks may lessen in severity with age
- Mortality has been significantly reduced by modern medical care
- Anticipate the risk of transmission in families with a history of the disorders
- Congenital myotonia results in no serious long-term sequelae except cramping

110. Thyrotoxic Myopathy

Etiology/Pathophysiology

- Thyrotoxic myopathy occurs in patients with significant hyperthyroidism
  - Thyrotoxicosis causes a shift in the expression of muscle toward fast-twitch fibers; muscle tension then occurs at lower calcium concentrations than usual
  - Increased rate of sarcoplasmic reticulum calcium uptake that disturbs energy metabolism
  - Combined accelerated metabolism and insulin resistance from thyrotoxicosis causes muscle energy depletion, and fatigability/weakness
  - Weakness occurs in as many 80% of thyrotoxic patients
  - Women more commonly affected than men, onset occurs in middle age
- Thyrotoxic periodic paralysis is characterized by acute attacks of weakness associated with hypokalemia (as in hypokalemic periodic paralysis) but occurs in thyrotoxic patients
  - Serum potassium is decreased during the attacks
  - Thyrotoxic states increase the number of Na-K pumps, possibly explaining the hyperkalemia and subsequent weakness as occurs with hypokalemia from other causes
  - Occurrence sporadic, frequently in Asians
  - See *Muscle Channelopathies*

Differential Dx

- Polymyositis
- Dermatomyositis
- Inherited myopathy
- Steroid myopathy
- Myasthenia gravis
- Guillain-Barré syndrome
- Amyotrophic lateral sclerosis
- Limb girdle muscular dystrophy

Presentation/Signs & Symptoms

- Thyrotoxic myopathy
  - Progressive proximal upper and lower extremity weakness
  - Preserved reflexes
  - Symptoms of hyperthyroidism (e.g., hyperpyrexia, diarrhea, weight loss, tachycardia)
  - Weakness out of proportion to visible muscle wasting
  - Coexistence of myasthenia gravis symptoms such as fluctuating diplopia or ptosis suggest presence of myasthenia gravis and thyrotoxicosis
- Thyrotoxic periodic paralysis: Abrupt onset of paralysis following high-carbohydrate meals or extreme exercise in thyrotoxic patients

Diagnostic Evaluation

- Thorough history to rule out exogenous steroid use and family history of periodic paralysis
- Serum potassium, thyroid function tests, and CK levels
- EMG and nerve conduction studies reveal a lack of neurogenic changes, demyelinating changes, or changes suggestive of amyotrophic lateral sclerosis
- Muscle biopsy will show similar findings as hypokalemic period paralysis with vacuolar myopathy representing increased sarcoplasmic reticulum diameter
  - Muscle biopsy is of little value if thyrotoxicosis is known to be present

Treatment/Management

- Management of thyrotoxicosis is the mainstay of treatment
  - Treatments include β-blockers, radioactive iodine ablation if Graves' disease is present, and use of thyroid-stimulating hormone inhibitors
- Cardiac monitoring may be necessary if severe tachycardia present

Prognosis/Complications

- Prognosis for both disorders is excellent with appropriate treatment
- Myocardial infarction and respiratory failure can occur if untreated

111. Intensive Care Neuromuscular Disorders

Etiology/Pathophysiology

- Proximal and/or distal symmetrical weakness is relatively common in patients confined to critical care setting for extended periods
  - Usually associated with excessive protein catabolism (e.g., sepsis, prolonged inactivity, neuromuscular blockade, corticosteroid exposure
- May be due to muscle disease (AQM) or nerve disease (CIP); many patients have features of both AQM and CIP
- AQM is generally described in patients requiring prolonged neuromuscular blockage with nondepolarizing muscle relaxants, which are often used to prevent agitation, and exposure to corticosteroids (e.g., classically occurs in COPD patients following exacerbations requiring oral steroids)
- CIP is classically seen in patients with sepsis with/without exposure to corticosteroids
- Physical inactivity is generally required for either syndrome secondary to activation of the atrogin-1 proteosome pathway, which is a final common pathway of muscle apoptosis
- In addition to physical inactivity, the catabolic state as seen in sepsis or induced by corticosteroid exposure accelerates the process

Differential Dx

- Myasthenia gravis
- Inflammatory myopathy
- Botulism
- Cervical myelopathy
- Rhabdomyolysis
- Guillain-Barré syndrome
- Brainstem stroke

Presentation/Signs & Symptoms

- Progressive symmetrical weakness, proximal greater than distal, in a patient in the catabolic state, generally in an ICU setting, many times associated with the use of chronic neuromuscular blocking agents and/or high-dose corticosteroids
- Often difficult to gauge onset as many of these patients are sedated and the neurological examination is clouded
- Cranial musculature is generally spared
- Pulmonary musculature may be involved, requiring ventilator dependence
- Reflexes preserved in AQM, absent in CIP
- Sensory loss always denotes CIP, but difficult to assess in the critical illness setting

Diagnostic Evaluation

- A high index of suspicion is necessary in patients on prolonged mechanical ventilation who are difficult to wean from mechanical ventilation or who do not move spontaneously
- EMG and NCS can help distinguish AQM from CIP in some cases; however, inability to move makes differentiating nerve and muscle disease difficult; some centers can directly stimulate muscle membrane and smaller nerves to distinguish CIP and AQM in some patients
- CSF analysis is normal
- Muscle biopsy with special staining for myosin may show a relative absence relative to actin, denoting AQM in the proper clinical setting
- Nerve biopsy is not specific for CIP
- CK level may be elevated early in AQM, although not usually over 1000

Treatment/Management

- No specific medication reverses either syndrome
- Minimize steroid use and neuromuscular blocking agents
- Treat the underlying syndrome (e.g., antibiotics for sepsis)
- Physical therapy

Prognosis/Complications

- Prognosis is generally excellent in cases of AQM, as long as the condition is not prolonged
- CIP generally occurs in patients with severe systemic inflammatory response syndromes and prolonged inactivity and carries a worse prognosis
- Patients who improve the most are those with COPD and those with minimal underlying pathologies that would require large continuous doses of neuromuscular blocking agents and steroids; they may improve from severe weakness to normal function within weeks
- Generally, mortality depends on the course of the underlying process with AQM/CIP as a marker of nerve and muscle cell apoptosis
- Inability to wean from mechanical ventilation may denote a longer course and poor outcome

Alterations in Consciousness

JON BRILLMAN, MD, FRCPI

Section 11

112. Coma

Etiology/Pathophysiology

- An alteration in consciousness caused by severe, bilateral hemispheric disease or damage to the ascending reticular activating system from the mid-pons through the thalamus
- Etiologies are numerous and include trauma, ischemic or anoxic encephalopathy, drugs and alcohol, endogenous metabolic abnormalities, vitamin deficiencies, subarachnoid hemorrhage, brainstem lesions (e.g., pontine stroke or hemorrhage), cerebellar mass, compression of the brainstem secondary to herniation of the temporal lobe from a supratentorial mass (e.g., subdural hematoma), psychogenic causes, and hypertensive hemorrhage with intraventricular extension
- Drowsiness is the first stage of coma; may appear asleep but respond to voice
- Stupor often then occurs, in which patients respond to pain but not to voice
- Coma is defined as no response to pain or voice
- Patient does not follow verbal commands, does not speak, and does not open eyes to pain (GCS score of ≤8)
- Decreased responsiveness despite an awake appearance may occur with bilateral prefrontal lesions (e.g., strokes, hemorrhages, tumors)

Differential Dx

- Hysterical unresponsiveness or psychogenic coma
- Sleep and/or oversedation, particularly in the elderly
- Nonconvulsive status epilepsy
- Frontal lobe tumors with abulia
- Persistent vegetative state due to bilateral hemisphere ischemia or anoxia
- "Locked-in" state secondary to pontine infarct

Presentation/Signs & Symptoms

- Pupillary abnormalities suggests etiology
  - A dilated, light-fixed pupil indicates temporal lobe herniation on the side of the pupillary abnormality with brainstem compression
  - Bilateral dilated, light-fixed pupils suggest hypoxia
  - Pinpoint pupils suggest opiate overdose, pontine infarction, or pontine hemorrhage
- Decerebrate posturing (hyperextension, rotation of arm, plantar flexion of leg) indicates brainstem lesion below midbrain
- Apneustic breathing (sustained inspiratory cramp), ataxic respirations (4–5/min), or hyperventilation may indicate brainstem disease

Diagnostic Evaluation

- Examination should include evaluation of brainstem functions, particularly pupillary responses and eye movements, respirations, and response to pain
- Eye movements determine whether coma is due to bilateral hemisphere disease or brainstem disease
  - Doll's head maneuver: Rotate head from side-to-side
  - Ice water calorics: 30 cc of ice water injected into ear; if eyes do not move, coma caused by brainstem disease; if eyes move slowly to side of ice water and then drift back to midline, coma is due to hemisphere disease
- Initial studies include blood and urine toxicology screen, chemistries, glucose, LFTs, TSH, ammonia, ECG, head CT
- CSF analysis if suspect hemorrhage and/or infection
- EEG is helpful to exclude subclinical status epilepsy or metabolic encephalopathy
- Cervical spine films if trauma along with imaging of brain to exclude subdural or epidural hematoma

Treatment/Management

- Intubation may be necessary for respiratory difficulty (usually medullary failure)
- Subdural and epidural hematoma requires neurosurgical intervention
- Seizures should be treated with IV phenytoin
- Narcan or naloxone should be administered if drug overdose is suspected
- IV thiamine should be administered if alcoholism or vitamin deficiency is suspected; should be given without glucose
- Correct any metabolic abnormalities
- Treat trauma appropriately

Prognosis/Complications

- Prognosis depends primarily on etiology
- In general, brainstem coma is a more serious than bihemispheric coma
- Structural disease usually carries a worse prognosis than metabolic disease, unless surgically correctable

113. Brain Death

Etiology/Pathophysiology

- Brain death is defined as complete cessation of all electrical activity of the cerebral hemispheres and brainstem
- Complete cessation of cerebral blood flow then occurs secondarily
- Carries the same legal status as cardiac death regarding termination of life

Differential Dx

- Hypothermia (below 91.4°F [33°C])
- Drug intoxication
- Deep coma

Presentation/Signs & Symptoms

- Apnea
- No response to deep pain
- Brainstem reflexes are absent, including pupillary responses, corneal reflexes, and response to tracheal stimulation
- Patient may have occasional "Lazarus reflexes," with elevation of an arm or tonic neck movements despite absence of cerebral and brainstem function

Diagnostic Evaluation

- Isoelectric EEG reveals electrocerebral silence
- The absence of cerebral blood flow can be evaluated with a nuclear scan, CTA, MRA, or transcranial Doppler
- Drug screening should be obtained to rule out intoxication
- Attempts should be made to identify the etiology of brain death, including blood screening and brain imaging
- Frequently, brain swelling with small ventricles and absent sulci is noted on CT or MRI
- Perform apneic oxygenation test
  - Obtain arterial blood gas and identify pCO_2
  - Terminate ventilator and allow patient to breath 100% oxygen via T-tube
  - pCO_2 will rise approximately 3 mmHg/min
  - After several minutes, if pCO_2 is above 55 mmHg and patient has not respired, this is evidence of brainstem death

Treatment/Management

- Discussion with family regarding nature of brain death
- Designation of organ(s) for transplant should be discussed with family, preferably prior to brain death

Prognosis/Complications

- If the above criteria are met, the patient may be declared legally dead and ventilator terminated

114. Persistent Vegetative State

Etiology/Pathophysiology

- A neurologic condition characterized by the absence of cortical function with preserved brainstem function
  - Patient appears awake but does not interact with environment
- Occurs due to incomplete resuscitation secondary to cardiac arrest, ischemic encephalopathy due to impaired cardiac output, respiratory failure, or terminal stages of dementia

Differential Dx

- Stupor or coma
- Postictal state
- Nonconvulsive status epilepsy
- Metabolic encephalopathy
- "Locked-in" state (pontine infarction)
- Psychogenic catatonia

Presentation/Signs & Symptoms

- Patient may have mouthing movements or grimacing
- Decorticate posturing with flexion of arms and hyperextension of legs
- Eyes may follow around the room
- The patient may swallow spontaneously but is not able to eat
- No interaction with environment
- No purposeful response to discomfort
- No ability to communicate

Diagnostic Evaluation

- EEG to evaluate for slowing and seizure activity
- Head CT scan or MRI to evaluate for structural lesions
- Metabolic screening and blood work, including drug screen
- Spinal fluid analysis may be indicated if suspect subarachnoid hemorrhage and/or infection

Treatment/Management

- Supportive care may include feeding tube and artificial ventilation in certain circumstances
- IV fluids

Prognosis/Complications

- Currently there are insufficient legal and ethical guidelines as to how to manage these patients
- Occasionally, young patients may recover after a prolonged period; however, adults in a persistent vegetative state do not recover after 1 wk
- A trial of extubation may be appropriate if the family agrees
- Discontinuation of feeding and fluids is extremely controversial and is still being assessed in courts on a case-by-case basis

115. Hypoxic-Ischemic Encephalopathy

Etiology/Pathophysiology

- An unfortunately common condition of (usually) irreversible brain damage caused by a critical reduction in cerebral blood flow or lack of oxygen to cerebral neurons
- Generally occurs secondary to cardiac arrest, ventricular arrhythmias, carbon monoxide poisoning, shock (either septic or hemorrhagic), drowning, choking, or respiratory failure from any cause
- Normally, cerebral blood flow is 55 mL/100 g of brain tissue per minute and is protected by autoregulation of blood flow; however, when the lower limit of the autoregulatory curve is exceeded for 5 min or when cerebral blood flow falls to <15 mL/100 g of brain tissue per minute, permanent necrosis of susceptible neurons occurs, including cortical neurons, basal ganglia neurons, thalamic cells, and Purkinje cells of the cerebellum (brainstem and spinal neurons are more resistant to damage)
- Anoxia or ischemia results in cellular edema and necrosis

Differential Dx

- Seizures and postictal state
- Hypoglycemic coma
- Traumatic brain injury
- Brainstem stroke or hemorrhage
- Cerebral hemorrhage
- Metabolic encephalopathy
- Drug intoxication
- Subarachnoid hemorrhage

Presentation/Signs & Symptoms

- Presentation depends on severity and length of hypoxia or ischemia
- Less than 5 min of insult may produce only confusion or agitation with mild memory failure upon recovery
- Greater than 5 min of anoxia results in stupor and coma
  - Apnea
  - Fixed, dilated pupils
  - Absent doll's head eye movements
  - Decerebrate or decorticate posturing
  - Bilateral Babinski signs
  - Reduction in deep tendon reflexes
  - Seizures (either generalized or myoclonic); may involve mouth or face

Diagnostic Evaluation

- History and physical examination including GCS
- Initial evaluation includes ECG, chest X-ray, arterial blood gas, CBC, and chemistries
- EEG may show slowing, seizure activity, or burst-suppression patterns (poor prognosis)
- Head CT scan or MRI are often normal but may show "watershed" infarcts in areas where blood supply is sparse or signs of generalized brain edema

Treatment/Management

- If resuscitative measures have failed and coma ensues, maintain airway and ventilation
- Steroids, calcium channel blockers, and glutamate antagonists are often used but have not been shown to be beneficial
- Cooling the patient (especially if febrile) has been shown in some studies to improve outcomes
- Anticonvulsant medication for seizures (e.g., phenytoin, benzodiazepines)
- A frank discussion with family members is necessary regarding prognosis and, in some cases, consideration of organ transplantation

Prognosis/Complications

- Mild cases without coma normally have full recovery, even if there is transient memory failure
- 80% mortality at 1 wk if patient presents in coma (see *Coma*)
- 20% may develop persistent vegetative states (see *Persistent Vegetative States*)

Neuro-Ophthalmology

JON BRILLMAN, MD, FRCPI
LARA J. KUNSCHNER, MD

116. Pupillary Abnormalities

Etiology/Pathophysiology

- Anisocoria is defined as unequal pupils
- Pupillary size represents an interplay between the sympathetic and parasympathetic nervous systems
- Pupils are more or less similar in size but may be 1 or 2 mm different and still be normal (essential anisocoria)
- Pupils tend to become smaller with advanced years
- Pupillary dilation (mydriasis) is effected by the action of the iris dilator muscle, which is under the control of the sympathetic system
  - Unopposed sympathetic activity by diminished parasympathetic action (e.g., CN III palsy) can cause anisocoria (abnormal pupil being larger), which is accentuated in light
  - Unilateral dilated pupil may be caused by mydriatic eye drops (atropine, scopolamine), postganglionic mydriasis (Adie's pupil), or preganglionic mydriasis (CN III palsy)
  - Bilateral dilated pupils may be due to glutethimide intoxication or anoxia
- Pupillary constriction (miosis) is effected by the action of the iris constrictor muscle, which is under parasympathetic control (CN III)
  - May be caused by cholinergic or parasympathomimetic drugs
  - If parasympathetic action is unopposed by sympathetic action (e.g., Horner's syndrome), anisocoria results and is more pronounced in dark

Differential Dx

- Medication or toxins causing pupillary dilation (e.g., anticholinergics, adrenergics, nicotine hallucinogens, MAO inhibitors)
- Medication or toxins causing pupillary constriction (e.g., opioids, cholinergics)
- Coma/anoxic encephalopathy
- Hippus (alternating sympathetic and parasympathetic tone)
- Horner's syndrome
- Compression of CN III nerve at skull base
- Adie's pupil
- Argyll-Robertson pupil

Presentation/Signs & Symptoms

- Normally a bright light will constrict pupils, directly and consensually
- There is normal alteration in sympathetic and parasympathetic tone with pupils becoming dilated and constricted alternately with sustained light stimulation (Hippus)
- Pupil should be checked for response to light and convergence
- Patients will complain of light intolerance due to impaired pupillary constriction
- Unilateral pupillary dilation in an awake patient is usually the result of mydriatic eye drops (atropine or scopolamine)

Diagnostic Evaluation

- Complete past medical and surgical history, with specific attention to neurologic, ophthalmologic, and head and neck region
- Physical examination should include measurement of pupil size in the light and the dark, pupil response to light and convergence, and lid position (especially with upgaze)
- In cases of third cranial nerve palsy, an MRI/MRA of the head may be indicated to rule out an aneurysm
- If Horner's syndrome is found, consider a chest CT to rule out apical lung mass (Pancoast tumor), MRI/MRA of head/neck, carotid Doppler, and/or carotid angiogram
- Place dilute pilocarpine drops to diagnose Adie's pupil

Treatment/Management

- Treat underlying disorder if possible
- Remove offending medications if possible
- Recommend eye protection (e.g., sunglasses) if photophobia occurs
- Adie's pupil is treated with pilocarpine drops for cosmesis and to aid in accommodation
- Treat migraines with triptans and/or pain medications for acute attacks and antidepressants, anticonvulsants, β-blockers, or calcium channel blockers to prevent further migraine episodes
- Neurosurgical evaluation of compressive lesions, structural lesions, tumors, masses, and aneurysms
- Narcotic overdose may be treated with naloxone

Prognosis/Complications

- Prognosis depends on the underlying etiology
- Horner's and Adie's syndromes are usually permanent
- Prognosis is favorable for compressive lesions that can be successfully removed; however, mydriasis may persist

117. Disorders of Eye Movements

Etiology/Pathophysiology

- Both CNS and PNS lesions can lead to disorders of either conjugate (bilateral) or isolated eye movement abnormalities resulting primarily in diplopia
- Most cases are due to strokes, multiple sclerosis, or vitamin deficiencies
- Central etiologies include progressive supranuclear palsy (paresis of voluntary gaze), Parkinson's disease (paresis of upgaze), strokes (conjugate gaze palsy or isolated ophthalmoparesis), multiple sclerosis (internuclear ophthalmoplegia), Wernicke's encephalopathy (paralysis of gaze or nystagmus)
- Peripheral etiologies include diabetic cranial neuropathy (CN III and VI), trauma (CN III, IV, and VI), myasthenia gravis (failure of neuromuscular transmission affecting any extraocular muscle)
- Upward gaze is damaged frequently by compression of tectum of the midbrain (e.g., Parinaud's syndrome) and involvement of the interstitial nucleus
- Horizontal eye movements are damaged either by isolated cranial nerve palsies of extraocular muscles, the parapontine reticular formation, or medial longitudinal fasciculus

Differential Dx

- Convergence spasm (hysteria)
- Drug intoxication including alcohol
- Fibrosis of the superior recti may be seen in advanced years in the absence of other disease
- Structural lesions of brainstem

Presentation/Signs & Symptoms

- Diplopia is the most common symptom
- Visual blurring
- Gaze deviation
- Pupils are most commonly involved with CN III palsies if lesion is compressive
- Paralysis of convergence seen in lesions of the midbrain
- "One and a half" syndrome is generally attributable to a stroke at the base of the pons involving parapontine reticular formation and ipsilateral medial longitudinal fasciculus; ipsilateral eye is totally paralyzed and contralateral eye has lateral deviation with nystagmus

Diagnostic Evaluation

- History, neurologic, and ocular examinations
  - Complete neurologic exam: Note focal neurologic deficits, cranial nerve involvement, cerebellar signs, and symptoms of demyelination (e.g., abnormal Romberg)
  - Ocular exam: Vision, pupil size and reaction, eye motility ductions and versions, ptosis, fundus exam, visual field defect, proptosis, and ice test (myasthenia gravis)
- If suspect CNS lesion, MRI is usually the test of choice
- CT is better for orbital etiologies (e.g., trauma, thyroid)
- MRI/MRA (and/or angiography) is indicated immediately in cases of pupil-involving CN III palsy, if age <50 (to rule out demyelinating disease), if no improvement over 3 mo, aberrant regeneration, multiple cranial nerve or systemic neurologic involvement exists
- CSF analysis if infection or neoplasm suspected
- Tensilon test (myasthenia gravis) and ESR (temporal arteritis) may be indicated

Treatment/Management

- Treat the underlying cause
- Eye patching is useful for diplopia
  - Patch one eye (usually the involved eye) as necessary
  - In children <10 y old, avoid patching and monitor for development of amblyopia
- Document magnitude of ocular deviation and/or diplopia to determine improvement or stability between exams (measured with prisms by ophthalmologist)
- Prisms may be included in glasses for small stable deviations
- Antiacetylcholinesterase medications and/or steroids for myasthenia gravis
- Thiamine supplementation for Wernicke's encephalopathy

Prognosis/Complications

- Ophthalmoparesis due to Wernicke's syndrome generally responds well to IV thiamine
- Diabetic ophthalmoparesis generally improves within 6–8 wk
- Internuclear ophthalmoplegia due to multiple sclerosis often improves spontaneously or with corticosteroids
- Myasthenic ophthalmoparesis generally responds well to treatment

118. Nystagmus

Etiology/Pathophysiology

- Nystagmus is an involuntary, rhythmic, biphasic oscillation of the eyes
- Characterized as horizontal, vertical, rotary, or a combination; fast or slow; symmetrical or asymmetrical; and pendular (equal speed in either direction) or jerk (slow in one direction followed by fast in the opposite direction)
- By convention, nystagmus is named in the direction of the fast phase
- Usually results from a defect in the slow eye movement system (visual fixation, vestibular system, smooth pursuit, vergence, optokinetic, and neural integrator pathways)
- May be normal or pathologic
- May be congenital or acquired
- Most cases of nystagmus are due to brainstem disorders, cranial nerve (especially CN VIII) disease, or cerebellar disease
- Horizontal nystagmus in extremes of gaze may be normal; otherwise, most often caused by drug intoxication (e.g., dilantin, barbiturates, benzodiazepines) or intramedullary brainstem disease
- Vertical upbeat nystagmus is seen in intrinsic brainstem disease (e.g., multiple sclerosis, stroke), rarely seen in drug intoxications
- Vertical downbeat nystagmus is commonly seen in lesions in the region of the foramen magnum (e.g., Arnold-Chiari malformation)
- Rotatory nystagmus is seen in central or peripheral vestibular disease

Differential Dx

- Non-nystagmus oscillations: Saccadic intrusions (e.g., square-wave jerks seen in cerebellar disease, ocular bobbing seen in brainstem infarcts, ocular dysmetria seen primarily in multiple sclerosis, opsoclonus/ myoclonus seen in paraneoplastic syndromes)
- Myasthenia gravis may cause nystagmus due to weakness of extraocular muscles

Presentation/Signs & Symptoms

- Oscillopsia (a sense that the surroundings are oscillating) may be present
- Vertigo may be present
- Diplopia may be present
- Disequilibrium may be present
- Associated symptoms may include nausea/vomiting, dysarthria, and ataxia

Diagnostic Evaluation

- Consider drug, toxin, and dietary screen of urine/serum
- MRI of brain may reveal tumors, demyelinating disease, vascular disease, and congenital malformations
- Consider eye movement recording or electronystagmogram (ENG), visual evoked responses, and electroretinography (ERG)
- In children with opsoclonus, an abdominal CT should be done to rule out neuroblastoma
- In adults, rule out paraneoplastic syndromes with anti-Ri antibodies and malignancy workup
- Workup for myasthenia gravis may be indicated

Treatment/Management

- Treat the underlying etiology if possible
- Remove offending medications/toxins if possible
- Medications to treat the nystagmus (e.g., meclizine) have varying success
- Congenital nystagmus: Maximize vision by refractive lenses, treat amblyopia ("lazy eye") if indicated, prism, and/or eye muscle surgery
- Vestibular nystagmus: Vestibular suppressant (meclizine, diazepam), vestibular adaptation exercises
- Baclofen may be useful in periodic alternating nystagmus and some congenital nystagmus
- Clonazepam for downbeat nystagmus

Prognosis/Complications

- Congenital nystagmus is not progressive
- Acquired nystagmus will generally resolve if underlying etiology is removed, but prognosis depends on the etiology

Etiology/Pathophysiology

- Vision loss may be unilateral or bilateral; transient or more persistent; of sudden or gradual onset; painless or painful
- Lesions can be localization to the retina, orbit, optic nerve or chiasm, optic radiations, occipital cortex, or visual association cortex
  - Retina: Detached retina, retinitis pigmentosa, macular degeneration
  - Orbital: Mass lesions, vitreous hemorrhage, corneal opacities
  - Optic nerve: Mass lesions, autoimmune/demyelination (e.g., optic neuritis), toxins, ischemia (e.g., embolism, temporal arteritis), carotid stenosis, giant cell arteritis, hyperviscosity, hypotension, severe disc edema, tobacco-alcohol amblyopia, optic atrophy, anterior ischemic optic neuropathy
  - Optic chiasm: Usually due to compressive mass lesions (e.g., pituitary adenoma, aneurysm, meningioma, craniopharyngioma)
  - Optic radiation: Mass lesions, ischemia, or intracerebral hemorrhage
  - Visual cortex: Unilateral visual loss may be due to mass lesions, vascular disease (e.g., ischemic stroke, intracranial hemorrhage, venous thrombosis, subarachnoid hemorrhage); bilateral transient visual loss may be due to migraine, vertebrobasilar insufficiency, prolonged hypertension or hypotension, drug-induced (e.g., cyclosporine toxicity), seizure, or postictal phenomenon

Differential Dx

- Hysteria/conversion disorder
- Transient obscurations (s) due to increased intracranial pressure
- Loss of vision (min) due to carotid or retinal ischemia
- Loss of vision (d) due to optic or retrobulbar neuritis
- Gradual and progressive loss of vision is often due to compressive lesions

Presentation/Signs & Symptoms

- Orbital: Blurring, black spots
- Optic nerve: Central scotoma, altitudinal defect, decreased acuity, often transient monocular visual loss (amaurosis fugax) if due to ischemia/embolism
- Optic chiasm: Bitemporal visual field abnormalities
- Optic tract: Incongruous hemianopsia contralateral to the lesion with normal acuity and papillary responses
- Visual cortex: Congruous homonymous hemianopsia contralateral to the lesion, if bilateral causes cortical blindness often with patient unaware of defect, may have "macular sparing" or small area of retained macular vision with good acuity, normal pupillary reactions

Diagnostic Evaluation

- Complete ophthalmological examination is necessary, possibly with fluorescein angiography
- Visual field testing
- MRI of brain and orbits with and without gadolinium
- Carotid duplex sonography and cardiac echocardiography if ischemia is considered
- Blood work analysis for vascular risk factors (e.g., lipids, coagulation screen, vasculitis screen, ESR)

Treatment/Management

- Corticosteroids are indicated for inflammatory, demyelinating, or vasculitic etiologies, including temporal arteritis
- Antiplatelet therapy and risk factor reduction for ischemic optic neuropathy or cortical stroke
- Consider carotid endarterectomy after transient monocular blindness if carotid stenosis greater than 70% is found in the carotid artery unilateral to the visual loss
- Neoplasms may warrant radiotherapy, resection, or no treatment

Prognosis/Complications

- In some situations, vision loss may be reversible with timely intervention
- Vision loss may be a harbinger of a more serious, even life-threatening conditions (e.g., brain tumor, meningitis, giant cell arteritis, cavernous sinus thrombosis, mucormycosis)
- Ischemic causes have poor prognosis for visual recovery
- Giant cell arteritis has high risk of involvement of the contralateral eye if not recognized and treated promptly with corticosteroids
- Optic neuritis associated with multiple sclerosis in 40–60% cases

Dizziness & Syncope

PATRICIA B. JOZEFCZYK, MD, FAAN

120. Lightheadedness

Etiology/Pathophysiology

- Lightheadedness is one of the most common symptoms in practice and prevalence increases with age
- The term is imprecise and may include symptoms of dizziness, vertigo, lightheadedness, presyncope, or disequilibrium
- Etiologies are numerous; most commonly caused by conditions that result in a relative decrease in cerebral perfusion
- Dizziness is more properly termed vertigo, which is a hallucination of movement, most typically spinning or rotational; etiologies include peripheral vestibular dysfunction or CNS disease
- Presyncope is a precise syndrome of lightheadedness associated with a graying of vision, tinnitus, and a realization that syncope is to follow; occurs secondary to cerebral hypoperfusion from decreased cardiac output or decreased peripheral vascular resistance
- Disequilibrium is a sense of imbalance that typically occurs when walking and can be due to problems with sensory proprioception or cerebellar system dysfunction
- Postural hypotension, cardiogenic factors, and defective vasopressor mechanisms are common in the elderly

Differential Dx

- Otologic etiologies (e.g., positional vertigo, Ménière's disease)
- CNS etiologies (e.g., vertebrobasilar ischemia, cerebellar or brainstem infarct, cerebellar hemorrhage, basilar migraine, cerebellar pontine angle tumor)
- Other systemic etiologies include arrhythmia, orthostatic hypotension, acute or chronic alcohol intoxication, salicylate toxicity, antiepileptic drug toxicity, uremia, diabetes, and thyroid disease
- Multiple medication use

Presentation/Signs & Symptoms

- Acute vertigo presents with severe rotational dizziness, nausea, vomiting, diaphoresis, and tachycardia
- Exam shows prominent nystagmus
    - Peripheral vestibular: Horizontal and unidirectional; often suppressed by visual fixation, produced by head rotation
    - Central: Horizontal or vertical; may be associated with skew deviation of eyes; not suppressed by fixation; may or may not be provoked by head rotation
- Otologic symptoms with vestibular causes (e.g., ear fullness, pain, tinnitus)
- CN signs (especially V and VII) or brainstem signs (e.g., facial/limb numbness, unilateral dysmetria) may occur with CNS disease

Diagnostic Evaluation

- Evaluation is guided by a detailed history, neurologic, otologic, and general physical examination
    - Orthostatic hypotension may be present
    - Should include the Hallpike-Dix maneuvers of head and neck rotation to elicit symptoms and nystagmus
- If a peripheral otologic source is suspected, evaluation should include audiogram with speech discrimination, posturography, ENG, caloric stimulation testing, or rotational chair testing
- If a CNS source is suspected, a CT scan or MRI of the brain with views of the posterior fossa, brainstem, and cerebellar pontine angle is indicated
- Systemic causes may be investigated with laboratory studies (CBC, chemistries, thyroid function tests, vitamin B_{12} level), ECG, cardiac Holter monitoring, orthostatic BP checks, and/or echocardiogram
- Tilt-table test may be used to identify orthostasis

Treatment/Management

- Acute peripheral vestibulopathy can be treated by vestibular suppressants, bed rest, and fluids; particle repositioning can be used for positional vertigo (modified Epley maneuver)
- Chronic peripheral vestibulopathy generally improves with vestibular rehabilitation; however, some persistent or progressive conditions (e.g., Ménière's disease, labyrinthine fistula) may require surgical intervention
- Central causes are not typically responsive to vestibular suppressant medication; treatment is aimed at management of the specific cause
- Systemic causes are also treated individually (e.g., antiarrhythmic agents or pacemaker for arrhythmias, fluids or intravascular volume expanders for orthostatic hypotension, adjustment in medications to limit drug-related dizziness)

Prognosis/Complications

- Prognosis depends on the underlying etiology
- Acute and episodic dizziness is typically short in duration with full recovery; some labyrinthine pathologies are recurrent and associated with hearing loss
- Chronic dizziness may persist if no treatment etiology is identified; this may progress with age
- Prognosis of CNS neoplasms depend on type, location, and size
- Degenerative neurologic diseases (e.g., spinocerebellar ataxia, Friedreich's ataxia) currently have no effective treatment

121. Syncope

Etiology/Pathophysiology

- A loss of consciousness secondary to inadequate cerebral perfusion
- Vasovagal syncope is the most common cause; this is a reflex syncope that results in bradycardia and hypotension; causes include carotid massage, micturition, valsalva, and situations resulting in a strong emotional response
- Decreased cerebral perfusion may occur with decreased cardiac output or decreased peripheral vascular resistance
    - Cardiac output can be decreased by arrhythmias, heart block, or cardiac arrest
    - Peripheral vascular resistance is decreased by medications or toxins (e.g., alcohol) that produce vasodilation
- Hypovolemia may also contribute to decreased cerebral perfusion; this may worsen with standing and result in orthostatic syncope
- In children, breath holding may result in syncope
- Postural hypotension is a common cause, especially in elderly populations

Differential Dx

- Seizure
- Vertebrobasilar stroke
- Complicated migraine
- Subarachnoid hemorrhage
- Cataplexy with narcolepsy
- Drop attacks from vertebrobasilar TIA
- Psychiatric pathology with conversion reaction

Presentation/Signs & Symptoms

- Loss of consciousness typically preceded by an awareness of impending syncope (presyncope), but may occur without warning in sudden cardiac events
- Presyncope includes lightheadedness, nausea, diaphoresis, tunneling or graying of vision, and muffled hearing or tinnitus
- When complete loss of consciousness follows, a fall to the ground occurs and there may be brief tonic-clonic or tonic-rigid extension of the limbs; the loss of consciousness is typically brief unless a persistent cardiac problem exists
- Cardiac syncope may be preceded by chest pain or palpitations
- Orthostatic syncope occurs with standing

Diagnostic Evaluation

- History and physical examination may be diagnostic
    - A history consistent with vasovagal syncope typically does not require further evaluation
    - Orthostatic BPs should be evaluated
    - Review of medications that may result in vasodilation (e.g., anticholinergics, tricyclic antidepressants, phenothiazines, antihypertensives)
- Suspected cardiac syncope should be evaluated with an ECG and Holter monitoring
- Hypovolemia may occur with anemia or electrolyte abnormalities
- EEG may be indicated if seizures are suspected

Treatment/Management

- Vasovagal syncope can be avoided by patient education; patients should be instructed to assume a recumbent position when presyncopal symptoms occur
- Discontinue medications that may provoke postural hypotension
- Cardiac syncope is managed by antiarrhythmic agents or pacemaker insertion
- Hypovolemia may respond to fluids, salt, and volume expanders
- Micturition syncope in males may be avoided by sitting on a commode

Prognosis/Complications

- Prognosis depends on the etiology
- Vasovagal syncope is more common in the young and may resolve over time
- Cardiogenic syncope should resolve once cardiac output is maintained
- Complications are related to injuries that may occur at the time of the fall

122. Hyperventilation Syndrome

Etiology/Pathophysiology

- A form of panic attack that is associated with overbreathing and metabolic changes (respiratory alkalosis)
- An abnormal reaction to anxiety or stress that produces a rapid respiratory rate
- Results in a respiratory alkalosis, which, along with the release of epinephrine, causes increased cerebrovascular resistance and decreased cerebral blood flow
- In this alkalotic setting, unbound calcium ions may be diminished, resulting in tetany
- More common in women

Differential Dx

- Metabolic acidosis may result in increased respiratory rate
- Primary pulmonary or cardiac disease that results in hyperventilation
- If loss of consciousness occurs, other causes of syncope should be considered
- Central neurogenic hyperventilation
- Panic attack

Presentation/Signs & Symptoms

- Anxiety is followed by increased rate of breathing and a subjective sense of shortness of breath
- Lightheadedness
- Tingling in the fingers and perioral area may occur
- Carpal-pedal spasm may occur
- If prolonged, loss of consciousness may ensue, including seizures

Diagnostic Evaluation

- History suggests the diagnosis
- Symptoms can be reproduced by voluntary hyperventilation
- Chest X-ray, ECG, and blood gases may be indicated in atypical cases

Treatment/Management

- Rebreathing into a paper bag reverses all symptoms
- Patient education to eliminate provoking causes
- Sedatives or psychiatric evaluation for recurrent anxiety or panic attacks

Prognosis/Complications

- No long-term complications

123. Benign Paroxysmal Positional Vertigo

Etiology/Pathophysiology

- A common cause of vestibular vertigo that is caused by particles that float freely in the posterior semicircular canal of the inner ear
- The canal becomes abnormally sensitive to gravity or linear acceleration, resulting in vertigo with position change
- This may be caused by a detached otoconia from the utricle or saccule or other debris (canalithiasis), which become free-floating in the endolymph of the posterior semicircular canal
- May follow an acute attack of vestibular neuronitis or labyrinthitis
- Frequent sequela of head trauma

Differential Dx

- Acoustic neuroma
- Vertebrobasilar insufficiency
- Cerebellar infarction
- Cerebellar hematoma
- Ménière's disease
- Basilar migraine
- Presyncope
- Orthostatic hypotension or disequilibrium

Presentation/Signs & Symptoms

- Acute spinning vertigo that occurs with change of position, most typically with head rotation, rolling over in bed, or neck hyperextension
- Onset is abrupt and lasts only a few minutes but may recur often
- May have been preceded by a more severe or prolonged episode of vertigo (e.g., labyrinthitis, vestibular neuronitis)
- Neurologic and otologic exam is normal, but nystagmus and symptoms may be reproduced with Hallpike-Dix maneuver

Diagnostic Evaluation

- History and physical examination are often diagnostic
  - Rotatory nystagmus is produced on Hallpike-Dix maneuver
- ENG reveals a decreased vestibular response on caloric stimulation
- Rotational testing shows directional preponderance
- Posturography shows a vestibular pattern
- Brain imaging may be necessary to exclude structural lesions
- Brainstem auditory provoked responses may help to localize the lesion

Treatment/Management

- Particle repositioning maneuvers (modified Epley maneuver) may resolve symptoms
- Habituating exercises are useful but may take several weeks to see effect
- Vestibular suppressant medication (e.g., meclizine) may help acutely but prolonged use may delay central vestibular compensation
- Vestibular rehabilitation
- Surgical section of the nerve to the posterior semicircular canal or plugging of the canal can be done for persistent symptoms that are unresponsive to conservative management

Prognosis/Complications

- Symptoms are usually self-limited
- Up to 75% of cases improve in several months, even without treatment
- Average duration of symptoms is 10 wk
- 25% continue to have symptoms for years if not treated
- Positional vertigo may recur years after the initial episode

124. Cerebellar Infarction

Etiology/Pathophysiology

- Infarction of the cerebellum, resulting in dizziness and disequilibrium
- Ischemic infarction may occur from atherosclerotic disease in the vertebrobasilar system, cardioembolic disease, or artery-to-artery embolus
  - Depending on the vessel involved, the infarction may occur in the cerebellum alone or in combination with a brainstem infarct
- Hemorrhagic infarction occurs secondary to hypertension, arteriovenous malformation, vascular tumors of the cerebellum (e.g., hemangioblastoma), or due to hemorrhagic transformation of an ischemic infarct

Differential Dx

- Benign positional vertigo
- Acute vestibular pathology (e.g., labyrinthitis)
- Subarachnoid hemorrhage
- Acute intoxication
- Meningitis
- Basilar migraine
- Acoustic neuroma

Presentation/Signs & Symptoms

- Abrupt onset of dizziness, ataxia of gait, dysmetria (inability to judge distances), nausea and vomiting, and headache
- Rapid decline of mental status may occur as pressure increases in the posterior fossa and brainstem is compressed; this is most typical with a hemorrhagic infarction or large ischemic infarcts
- Other brainstem signs include cranial nerve palsies and Horner's syndrome
- As brainstem compression progresses, BP may be elevated and bradycardia may occur; breathing abnormalities may range from hyperventilation to Cheyne-Stokes respirations and apneustic respirations

Diagnostic Evaluation

- Cerebellar infarction is a medical emergency that requires emergent neuroimaging
- CT scan without contrast will identify a cerebellar hemorrhage and may show early ischemic patterns
- Toxicology screen to rule out acute intoxication that mimics brainstem or cerebellar disease
- Lumbar puncture should not be performed unless infection is suspected and CT scan is normal
- MRA may be indicated to evaluate the integrity of the posterior circulation

Treatment/Management

- Intubation if necessary to maintain airway
- Stabilization of BP
- Acute treatment is often unnecessary
- Antiplatelet medication may be indicated in ischemic events
- If brainstem compression is occurring, surgical decompression of the hemorrhage or ischemic cerebellar hemisphere may be indicated

Prognosis/Complications

- Death may occur from brainstem compression
- Survivors may have residual cerebellar or brainstem deficits (e.g., persistent gait instability, clumsiness, ophthalmoparesis)
- If unilateral cerebellar hemisphere is infarcted or removed surgically, the dysmetria and ataxia may improve over time as the brain adapts

125. Ménière's Disease

Etiology/Pathophysiology

- A disease of the inner ear caused by an accumulation of fluid (hydrops), resulting in severe vertigo
- Also results in degeneration of cochlear hair cells as the disease progresses, resulting in progressive deafness and tinnitus
- Cause is unknown; there may be a heritable component
- Onset usually in mid-life

Differential Dx

- Benign positional vertigo
- Labyrinthitis
- Brainstem infarct or TIA
- Cerebellar infarct
- Acoustic neuroma

Presentation/Signs & Symptoms

- Abrupt attacks of vertigo lasting several minutes or hours
    - Attacks are intermittent and random
- Unilateral deafness
    - With each attack of vertigo, deafness gets worse
    - After each attack, deafness and vertigo subside but successive attacks lead to permanent deafness
- Constant, low-pitched, unilateral tinnitus
- Fullness in ear
- Nausea and vomiting
- Rotatory nystagmus
- Past-pointing may occur during attack
- Sudden falls

Diagnostic Evaluation

- History and physical examination including Weber and Rinné tests and speech discrimination
- Audiometrics to evaluate for hearing loss
- Brainstem auditory evoked responses to evaluate the location of hearing loss
- Electronystagmography is used to determine a peripheral versus central lesion

Treatment/Management

- Initial treatments to reduce excess fluid in the ear include bed rest, salt restriction, and diuretics
- Avoidance of alcohol has been shown to be useful
- Meclizine or scopolamine patches act as a vestibular suppressant to reduce vertigo
- Antiemetics for symptomatic relief of nausea and vomiting
- Surgical destruction of the labyrinth may be attempted in intractable cases

Prognosis/Complications

- Permanent deafness occurs in 20% of patients
- Attacks tend to recur but usually stabilize after a few years with therapy and may remit entirely

Back Pain, Neck Pain, Spinal Cord & Nerve Root Disorders

PATRICIA B. JOZEFCZYK, MD, FAAN

126. Low Back Pain

Etiology/Pathophysiology

- An extremely common complaint that affects 80% of the population at some time in their lives
- May be caused by bone, joint, muscle, ligament, or nerve disease
- The functional spinal unit consists of vertebral body, intervertebral disc, facet joints, and associated ligamentous tissues; these units are responsible for spinal movement
- Arthritic causes: Osteoarthritis/degenerative joint (or disc) disease, rheumatoid arthritis, spondyloarthropathies
- Mechanical causes: Disk/facet disease, spondylolisthesis, fractures
- Postural causes: Osteoporosis and poor posture (excessive demands on back musculature cause lactic acid buildup and pain)
- Myofascial causes: Muscle/ligament strain, fascial tension, fibromyalgia
- Other serious causes: Spinal stenosis, cauda equina syndrome, infection (e.g., osteomyelitis or epidural abscess), and malignancy (especially prostate, breast, lung mets or myeloma)
- Red flags that may signal a serious cause of LBP (imaging should be strongly considered in these cases): Age >50 or <20, trauma, fever, abnormal neuro exam, worse pain at night/rest, known malignancy, immunosuppression, bowel/bladder dysfunction, and anticoagulation use

Differential Dx

- Mechanical low back pain
- Discogenic disease
- Systemic arthritides (RA, ankylosing spondylitis)
- Sacroiliitis
- Spinal stenosis
- Congenital spine malformations (e.g., occult spina bifida, spondylolisthesis)
- Neoplasms of vertebrae
- Osteomyelitis or discitis
- Lesions of conus medullaris or cauda equina
- Referred pain (AAA, PUD, pancreatitis, renal colic, endocarditis, UTI, prostatitis)

Presentation/Signs & Symptoms

- Pain from lumbar sprain/strain may localize to back or radiate to hips, coccyx, and upper leg
- Pain that radiates into lower leg suggests lumbar radiculopathy or disk disease
- Low back tenderness may be present and paraspinal muscle spasm may be palpable
- Limited lumbar range of motion
- Pain, fever, and/or pain with percussion over the posterior spinous processes suggests infection or neoplasm
- Straight leg raise test is positive for diskogenic or radicular pain
- Scoliosis may be present
- Antalgic gait

Diagnostic Evaluation

- History and physical are often diagnostic
- Imaging (MRI or CT myelogram) is indicated in patients with evidence of cord compression, red flag symptoms, or suspicion of epidural abscess or osteomyelitis
    - MRI is the study of choice: Visualizes soft tissue and spinal canal; can rule out malignancy, epidural abscess, osteomyelitis, cord compression, cauda equina syndrome, disk herniation, and nerve root compression
    - CT will only visualize bone (obtain CT myelogram to visualize cord/canal in patients unable to undergo MRI)
- X-rays of the lumbar spine are of little value unless trauma has occurred or a congenital abnormality is suspected
- Bone scan is helpful if infection or metastatic disease suspected
- Abdominal scan if pelvic or organ pathology suspected
- Gynecological examination and urinalysis in selected cases

Treatment/Management

- Conservative treatment is sufficient for patients without red flag symptoms
    - Return to activity as soon as possible; rest has not been shown to improve recovery
    - Acetaminophen, NSAIDs, opioids, and muscle relaxants for pain
    - Educate patient on proper biomechanics/ergonomics
    - Physical therapy, including pain relief modalities (e.g., ice, heat, ultrasound), stretching, strengthening, aerobic conditioning, and relaxation techniques
- Surgery may be considered in cases of refractory disease, large neurologic deficits, unbearable pain, or significant limitations

Prognosis/Complications

- Precise diagnosis is often never determined
- More than 90% of patients with acute mechanical low back pain return to baseline in 2–8 wk with conservative management
- Pain lasting more than 4–6 wk may indicate the need for imaging
- Psychiatric intervention may be indicated, including for cases involving workers' compensation or litigation

127. Lumbar Radiculopathy

Etiology/Pathophysiology

- Also known as sciatica
  - An extremely common disorder; usually due to a posterolateral lumbar disk herniation that irritates and compresses its associated nerve root
  - Lesion generally occurs as the nerve exits the spinal canal through the neural foramen
  - The nerve root can also be compromised in the lumbar plexus within the retroperitoneal space or distally in the sciatic notch
- May rarely be due to direct compression from an osteophyte or from sterile (noninfectious) inflammation
- Most commonly involves the L5 and S1 nerve roots
- L4 radiculopathy results in pain in the hip and anterior thigh to the knee; sensory change occurs in the anterior thigh or groin; weakness of the knee extensors and decreases patellar reflex
- L5 radiculopathy results in pain in the posterolateral thigh and dorsal foot; the lateral calf or large toe may have sensory loss; weakness of the extensor hallucis longus or ankle dorsiflexors may be present
- S1 radiculopathy results in pain in the posterolateral thigh, calf, and plantar surface of the foot; sensory change is noted in the lateral calf and lateral toes; weakness of plantar flexion and decreased Achilles reflex

Differential Dx

- Muscular strain
- Degenerative joint or disk disease
- Diabetic mononeuritis
- Herpes-zoster neuropathy
- Meralgia paresthetica (compression of the lateral femoral cutaneous nerve)
- Peroneal neuropathy
- Neuroma (e.g., Morton's neuroma, Joplin's neuroma)
- Lumbar plexus compression/infiltration
- Cauda equina tumors

Presentation/Signs & Symptoms

- Lower extremity pain (especially below the knee) is the most common symptom
  - Pain may be present in the back or buttocks and radiate into the leg
  - Pain is improved when lying supine and worsened when standing, sitting, or with valsalva (e.g., cough), which increases intraspinal pressure
- Straight leg raise may reproduce pain if the L5 or S1 nerve roots are involved
- Reverse straight leg raise may reproduce pain if the L3 or L4 nerve roots are involved
- Pain, paresthesias, motor deficit, and reflex changes may occur in the leg, depending on the nerve root involved

Diagnostic Evaluation

- History and physical examination is often diagnostic
- X-rays of the lumbar spine are of little value unless trauma has occurred or metastatic disease is suspected
- MRI will confirm the presence of a herniated disk, neural foramen compromise, malignancy, infection, and other pathologies
  - CT scan with myelogram may be used for patients who cannot undergo MRI or if MRI is equivocal
- EMG and nerve conduction studies may demonstrate nerve root dysfunction or muscle denervation
  - May also be used to distinguish between a lumbar plexus lesion versus a nerve root lesion as paraspinal muscles are involved in nerve root lesions but not plexus lesions
- Pelvic CT scan may be indicated in some cases if retroperitoneal disease or hemorrhage is considered

Treatment/Management

- Acute radiculopathy is most commonly managed conservatively with bed rest, analgesics, and muscle relaxants
- Steroids or NSAIDs may be useful
- Traction is of little benefit
- Physical therapy
- Surgical decompression (diskectomy) may be necessary if pain is unresponsive to conservative management or if there is progression of muscular weakness

Prognosis/Complications

- Prognosis is good when symptoms of pain and paresthesias respond to conservative treatment
- Depending on duration of nerve root compression, muscle weakness or reflex changes may be permanent
- There is an increased risk of recurrent disk herniation

128. Lumbar Spinal Stenosis

Etiology/Pathophysiology

- A condition involving the lower extremities that is often associated with degenerative disk and bone disease in the lumbar spine
- Most often due to degenerative arthritis with hypertrophy of the facet joints and supporting ligaments, resulting in gradual narrowing of the lumbar spinal canal with cord compression or nerve root impingement
- Results in compression of multiple nerve roots and claudication to the radicular arteries
- Lumbar nerve roots and the radicular arteries that travel with the nerve roots are compressed by osteophytes, hypertrophied ligamentum flavum, and protruding disks at several levels, most commonly L3-4, L4-5, and L5-S1
- Most common in elderly patients and athletes who have suffered multiple traumatic injuries
- Also often seen in patients who have had lumbar discectomy surgery
- Most commonly seen after sixth decade of life
- Known as pseudoclaudication, because symptoms imitate those of vascular claudication
  - Vascular claudication (i.e., peripheral vascular disease) generally presents with unilateral symptoms; spinal stenosis presents with bilateral symptoms

Differential Dx

- Intermittent claudication due to arterial disease
- Lumbar disk herniation
- Cauda equina syndrome due to meningeal cancer
- Arthritis of spine
- Compression fractures of spine
- Lumbar plexus syndrome
- Synovial cyst
- Tumor

Presentation/Signs & Symptoms

- Symptoms are generally exacerbated by exertion and relieved by rest and lumbar flexion
- Low back pain
- Scattered bilateral leg pain and numbness, especially occurring with exercise
- Weakness in legs, especially with exercise
- Leg pain with orthostasis
- Loss of knee or ankle reflexes
- Foot drop with walking
- Inability to climb hills
- Bladder or bowel symptoms are rarely present

Diagnostic Evaluation

- Plain films of lumbar spine are generally not useful unless trauma has occurred
- MRI of lumbar spine with and without enhancement will identify 90% of cases
- CT myelogram if unable to undergo MRI (e.g., too large to fit in MRI machine, claustrophobia)
- EMG and nerve conduction studies of the lower extremities will identify nerve root involvement
- Arterial Doppler ultrasound of the lower extremities may be indicated to differentiate spinal stenosis from vascular claudication

Treatment/Management

- NSAIDs and epidural steroid injections are the initial treatments
- Physical therapy, including back exercises, moist heat, and ultrasound
- Surgery (lumbar decompression) may be indicated if conservative medical management fails or if significant neurologic symptoms or signs are present
  - Epidural steroid injections, when started before surgery, have been shown to improve outcomes

Prognosis/Complications

- More than 60% of cases have symptomatic relief with conservative medical management
- Of those who undergo surgery, greater than 80% will have adequate symptom relief
- Preexisting neurologic deficits rarely improve with surgery; however, surgical correction will markedly lessen the chance of significant progression
- Potential complications of surgery include infection, CSF leakage, and new or worsened neurologic deficits (e.g., numbness, weakness, paralysis, pain, bowel/bladder dysfunction)

129. Cervical Radiculopathy

Etiology/Pathophysiology

- An extremely common disorder of middle-aged adults
- An irritation of a cervical nerve root that results in radiating pain, paresthesias, and weakness of the upper extremity
- Most commonly due to disk herniation or osteophyte that compresses the nerve root in the neural foramen
- C8 radiculopathy results in pain in the ulnar forearm and hand; numbness in the medial forearm and small finger; weakness may occur in the intrinsic hand muscles, finger flexors, and wrist extensors
- C7 nerve root disease is the most common cervical radiculopathy (70% of cases); results in pain in the posterolateral upper arm and shoulder; numbness in the index and middle fingers; weakness of the wrist flexors, finger extensors, and triceps; the triceps reflex is decreased
- C6 radiculopathy (20% of cases) results in pain in the shoulder, upper arm, lateral forearm, and thumb; numbness occurs in the lateral forearm, thumb, and index finger; weakness occurs in the biceps and wrist extensors; the biceps and brachioradialis reflex are decreased
- C5 radiculopathy results in pain in the shoulder and lateral upper arm, numbness of the shoulder area, and weakness in the deltoid and biceps; biceps reflex is decreased
- C4 is uncommon and results in shoulder pain and deltoid muscle weakness

Differential Dx

- Nondiskogenic cervical sprain or strain
- Arthritis of the cervical spine or shoulder
- Compression fracture of a vertebral body
- Rheumatoid arthritis
- Congenital abnormalities of skull base (e.g., basilar invagination, platybasia)
- Brachial plexopathy, carpal tunnel syndrome, or neuropathy
- Neoplasm or infection of vertebrae or disk space
- Rotator cuff injury
- Carotid or vertebral artery dissection
- Cardiac ischemia/infarct
- Tendonitis of the elbow

Presentation/Signs & Symptoms

- Neck pain with radiation to the arm in a dermatomal distribution
- Pain may increase with specific neck positions that further compromise the nerve root
- Pain, paresthesias, muscle weakness, and reflex changes occur in the distribution of the involved dermatome
- Reflex muscle spasm may occur secondarily causing localized pain
- Decreased cervical range of motion, especially of rotation and lateral flexion
- If there is associated cord compression, myelopathic signs may include gait disturbance, leg weakness, spasticity, and sphincter dysfunction
- Horner's syndrome may rarely occur

Diagnostic Evaluation

- Clinical presentation is often diagnostic
- X-rays of the cervical spine may reveal osteophytes, neural foramen encroachment, or decreased height of disk spaces
  - The base of the skull can also be visualized to evaluate for congenital bone abnormalities
- MRI is the best diagnostic modality to identify disk herniation or nerve root compression
  - CT with myelogram may also be used
- EMG (may not be positive for up to 2 wk) and nerve conduction studies may show nerve root dysfunction and muscle denervation

Treatment/Management

- Acute radiculopathy can be managed conservatively in 50% of cases with bed rest, analgesics, and muscle relaxants
- Steroids or NSAIDs may relieve symptoms
- Traction is often helpful, as is temporary immobilization with a soft collar
- Physical therapy modalities hasten recovery
- Surgical decompression of the nerve root with spinal fusion surgery may be necessary if pain is unresponsive to conservative management or if there is progression of muscular weakness

Prognosis/Complications

- Prognosis is good when symptoms of pain and paresthesias respond to conservative treatment
- Depending on duration of nerve root compression, muscle weakness or reflex changes may be permanent
- There is an increased risk of recurrent disk herniation in adjacent levels after surgical disk fusion
- If myelopathy is present, signs of cord compromise may be permanent

130. Cervical Spondylotic Myelopathy

Etiology/Pathophysiology

- The most common cause of spinal cord disease in adults
- Most often due to degenerative arthritis with hypertrophy of the facet joints and supporting ligaments, resulting in gradual narrowing of the cervical spinal canal with compression of the spinal cord or nerve root impingement
- Primarily occurs due to the natural aging process or repeated trauma; may be seen following cervical surgery
- Most commonly seen after sixth decade of life
- Vascular compromise as well as direct compression may occur
- Some individuals have a congenitally narrowed canal and are at increased risk for symptomatic disease and myelopathy

Differential Dx

- Amyotrophic lateral sclerosis
- Syringomyelia
- Multiple sclerosis
- Arteriovenous malformation of the spinal cord
- Acute transverse myelitis
- AIDS myelitis
- Tumor

Presentation/Signs & Symptoms

- Neck pain and bilateral arm pain
- Gait abnormalities (spastic-ataxic gait)
- Lhermitte's phenomena (paresthesias in back, buttocks, or legs on neck flexion)
- Clumsiness of hands
- Intrinsic hand muscle atrophy with fasciculations in advanced cases
- Myelopathy with pathological reflexes (hyperreflexia)
- Numbness or paresthesias of the lower extremities, which may ascend
- Loss of position sense and impaired vibratory sense in feet
- Babinski signs
- Sensory level in the cervical area
- Urinary urgency may occur late

Diagnostic Evaluation

- MRI of the cervical spine will identify 90% of cases
- CT myelogram in patients who are unable to undergo MRI (e.g., too large to fit in MRI machine, claustrophobia)
- EMG and nerve conduction velocity studies are not useful because the nerve roots are not affected

Treatment/Management

- NSAIDs and epidural steroid injections are the initial treatments
- Physical therapy with cervical traction
- Antispastic drugs (e.g., Lioresal)
- Bladder suppressants (e.g., tolterodine)
- Surgery (cervical decompression) may be indicated if conservative medical management fails or if significant neurologic symptoms or signs are present
  - Epidural steroid injections, when started before surgery, have been shown to improve outcomes

Prognosis/Complications

- Often progressive
- More than 60% of cases will have symptomatic relief with conservative medical management
- Of those who undergo surgery, >80% will have adequate symptom relief; however, surgery may play a greater role in preventing progression of disease or catastrophic events (e.g., quadriplegia)
- Preexisting neurologic deficits rarely improve with surgery; however, surgical correction will markedly lessen the chance of significant progression
- Potential complications of surgery include infection, CSF leakage, and new or worsened neurologic deficits (e.g., numbness, weakness, paralysis, pain, bowel/bladder dysfunction)
- Quadriplegia may occur with sudden neck injuries, such as whiplash

131. Acute Paralytic Brachial Neuropathy

Etiology/Pathophysiology

- Also known as Parsonage-Turner syndrome
- An inflammatory condition of the brachial plexus that results in pain and weakness in the upper arm
- The brachial plexus is the area in the region of the axilla where the cervical nerve roots merge to form the individual nerves that supply the arm
- The exact cause is unknown; most cases are idiopathic and may involve any part of the brachial plexus
  - Autoimmune reaction or infectious agent has been suggested as the etiology
  - There have been small epidemics in military personnel and cases reported after IV heroin use
  - Postimmunization cases have also been reported
- Men are more often affected than women
- Typically unilateral, but occurs bilaterally in up to 30% of cases

Differential Dx

- Trauma or avulsion of the brachial plexus
- Metastatic disease may compress or infiltrate the plexus (e.g., breast cancer)
- Radiation plexopathy
- Thoracic outlet syndrome
- Regional pain syndrome (typically follows limb surgery or injury)
- Entrapment neuropathies of the suprascapular or long thoracic nerves
- Adhesive capsulitis ("frozen shoulder syndrome")
- Amyotrophic lateral sclerosis

Presentation/Signs & Symptoms

- Acute onset of pain around the shoulder, which may radiate to the neck and arm
- Within a few days, weakness and sensory loss occurs in the arm, associated with loss of muscle stretch reflexes
- Unilateral involvement is most common
- Muscle weakness may be profound and is followed rapidly by muscle atrophy
- An upper trunk lesion resulting in C5-6 signs is the most common injury pattern and results in loss of voluntary control of the shoulder and elbow
- The whole plexus may be involved, resulting in a flail arm

Diagnostic Evaluation

- Diagnosis is made by the classic clinical presentation
- EMG and nerve conduction studies show motor and sensory involvement with an axonal neuropathy with some denervation characteristics
  - The distribution of abnormalities depends on the part of the plexus involved
  - Occasional widespread nerve conduction slowing is noted, implying a systemic disorder
- X-ray or MRI of the cervical spine, chest, and shoulder is indicated in atypical cases to rule out nerve root disease or masses that may compress the plexus
- MRI of the brachial plexus may be indicated if compression or metastatic disease is suspected
- CSF analysis is generally not necessary but will reveal elevated protein

Treatment/Management

- A 7–14 d course of steroids is generally the initial treatment
- Immobilization of the arm and shoulder may provide symptomatic relief
- Analgesics, including narcotics, may be necessary
- Physical therapy should be started once acute pain resolves

Prognosis/Complications

- Prognosis depends on the severity of the initial insult
- 65% of cases result in a good prognosis
- 15% of cases have poor results and 20% have a fair chance of recovery
- Even with intense therapy, recovery may take up to 3 y

132. Herpes-Zoster Neuropathy

Etiology/Pathophysiology

- Also known as shingles
- An inflammation of nerve roots (usually thoracic) caused by reactivation of herpes zoster virus
- Varicella zoster infection ("chicken pox") initially occurs, usually in childhood; the herpesvirus then lies dormant in dorsal root ganglia until reactivation occurs, usually secondary to physiologic stress, old age, or immunosuppression
- There is lymphocytic infiltration and inflammation of the affected nerve ganglia and may extend to the meninges and nerve root entry zone where the dorsal root enters the spinal cord
- A common disorder with an incidence of 1–5 per 1000 patients per year
    - Incidence is higher in patients with malignancies or immunocompromise
- More common in middle-aged adults and the elderly
- May occur in spinal or cranial ganglia
    - Geniculate (cranial nerve VII) zoster results in eruption on the tympanic membrane and in the external auditory canal and may cause facial paralysis (Ramsay Hunt syndrome)
    - Cranial nerve V eruptions result in ophthalmic zoster and ophthalmitis; extraocular muscle palsy may occur

Differential Dx

- Disease of the abdomen or thorax (e.g., appendicitis, myocardial ischemia)
- Cervical or lumbar radiculopathy
- Diabetic mononeuropathy
- Geniculate ganglion (cranial nerve VII) involvement may mimic Bell's palsy
- Meningitis should be considered if meningeal signs and headache are present

Presentation/Signs & Symptoms

- Pain and dysesthesia (extreme sensitivity to touch) initially occur in the distribution of affected nerve root; usually confined to the contiguous roots
- After 3–4 d, reddening of the skin occurs and vesicles appear in clusters in a dermatomal distribution; vesicles have clear fluid and may coalesce
- In 10–14 d, the vesicles scab and desquamate, leaving a pigmented scar
- Painless lymphadenopathy may occur
- Muscle weakness followed by atrophy may occur in a dermatomal distribution
- Fever, malaise, headache, confusion, and stiff neck may occur
- 80% of eruptions occur in the spinal ganglia (thoracic most common)

Diagnostic Evaluation

- The typical rash occurring in a dermatomal distribution confirms the diagnosis
- Vesicular fluid may be evaluated by electron microscopy or immunohistological staining for viral identification
- CSF analysis may reveal lymphocytic pleocytosis and elevated protein
    - CSF abnormalities are common with cranial ganglia involvement but less common with thoracic zoster and single segment zoster

Treatment/Management

- No treatment is available to prevent a zoster outbreak
- Acute zoster is treated with analgesics
- Oral corticosteroids are used to prevent postherpetic neuralgia
- Antiviral drugs (e.g., acyclovir, vidarabine) may decrease pain, decrease viral shedding, and increase healing but do not prevent postherpetic neuralgia
- IV antiviral agents should be used in immunocompromised patients or those who develop encephalitis or arteritis
- Postherpetic neuralgia may be treated with gabapentin or tricyclic antidepressants

Prognosis/Complications

- Acute zoster eruption may be associated with a myelitis or encephalitis from direct viral involvement
- Polyneuritis is less common
- Arteritis of the carotids may occur with ophthalmic zoster and can cause a contralateral hemiplegia that occurs from weeks to months after the acute infection
- Postherpetic neuralgia is the most common sequelae
    - Results in persistent sharp and shooting pains and dysesthesias
    - May persist for months or years and may be refractory to treatment
    - More common in elderly patients with ophthalmic or thoracic zoster

133. Winged Scapula

Etiology/Pathophysiology

- An unstable scapula due to failure of fixation against the posterior chest wall secondary to dysfunction of one or more of the scapular muscles
- Although direct muscle weakness or injury may be the etiology, most commonly this is due to an underlying nerve lesion of those nerves that supply the scapular muscles, including the long thoracic nerve, spinal accessory nerve, or dorsal scapular nerve
  - The long thoracic nerve innervates the serratus anterior muscle, which stabilizes the shoulder in abduction of the arm and holds the scapula flat against the back by keeping the inner margin fixed to the thorax; may be injured by direct pressure or trauma
  - The spinal accessory nerve innervates the upper fibers of the trapezius muscle, which pulls the scapula upward; may be injured by surgical procedures or direct trauma
  - The dorsal scapular nerve innervates the rhomboid muscles and is rarely involved in isolation
- Nerve lesions may occur from pressure on the shoulder, stab wounds, improper use of crutches, surgery, or tumors

Differential Dx

- Cervical radiculopathy
- Brachial plexopathy
- Mononeuritis multiplex

Presentation/Signs & Symptoms

- Winging of the medial border of the scapula or medial rotation of the inferior angle of the scapula
- Observation of the scapula position at rest and with specific movements helps to localize the involved nerve
- In long thoracic nerve lesions, the superior angle of the scapula is displaced medially and the inferior angle swings laterally; extending the arm in front of the body will accentuate winging
- In spinal accessory lesions, the upper vertebral border of the scapula moves away from the vertebrae while the lower angle remains relatively fixed and the shoulder is depressed; abduction of the arm will accentuate winging

Diagnostic Evaluation

- History and physical examination are helpful
- EMG and nerve conduction studies confirm the involved nerve
- MRI of the neck may be indicated to exclude a neoplasm if no obvious trauma or surgery is present

Treatment/Management

- Treatment of the underlying cause
- Stretch or pressure injuries may improve with time and physical therapy

Prognosis/Complications

- Stretch injuries may recover partially or fully with time
- Surgical injuries or trauma that results in severe nerve injury or transection may result in permanent muscle weakness

Sleep Disorders

Section 15

JAMES P. VALERIANO, MD

134. Insomnia

Etiology/Pathophysiology

- Difficulty falling asleep and/or frequent awakenings
- Insomnia may be a primary diagnosis or a symptom secondary to an underlying acute or chronic systemic or neuropsychiatric disorder
- Affects up to 40% of the U.S. population
- Acute, transient insomnia (<4 wk) may be due to situational stress, acute illness or injury, medications/drugs (e.g., cocaine, caffeine, ephedrine), changes in sleep environment, or reactive depression
- Chronic insomnia generally begins in early childhood and is lifelong
  - Difficulty falling asleep: Poor sleep hygiene, conditioned insomnia (maladaptive distorted sleep cognitions), medications (e.g., sedatives, decongestants, oral contraceptive use, antidepressants, bronchodilators), drugs (including over-the-counter and herbal preparations, alcohol, nicotine, illicit drugs), and caffeine (e.g., coffee, soda, medications)
  - Difficulty staying asleep: Sleep apnea, medications/drugs (e.g., alcohol), depression, anxiety, dementia, psychosis, mania, posttraumatic stress disorder, and various medical conditions (e.g., COPD, asthma, CHF, arrhythmias, angina, GERD, PUD, IBD, BPH, UTI, pregnancy, uremia, DM, hyperthyroidism, menopause, pain, pruritus, seizures)
- Movement disorder: Periodic movements of sleep, myoclonus, restless legs

Differential Dx

- Other causes of daytime hypersomnolence
  - Obstructive sleep apnea
  - Inadequate sleep time
  - Fictitious insomnia
  - Normal sleep time by polysomnogram

Presentation/Signs & Symptoms

- Daytime hypersomnolence
- Irritability
- Inability to sleep
- Mood disorders
- Decreased memory
- Decreased attention span
- Decreased job/school performance

Diagnostic Evaluation

- Careful history and physical examination are paramount
  - Many patients have insomnia but do not tell their doctors; ask questions about sleep quality during health maintenance visits
  - Note sleep habits, time spent in bed or trying to sleep elsewhere, bed mate, noise, safety, and interruptions
  - Medication/drug history
- Sleep diary is the most effective specific assessment tool
  - Should be recorded each morning
  - Include time in bed, time asleep, awakenings, quality of sleep, other symptoms (pain, dyspnea, urinary frequency)
- Polysomnography to evaluate sleep apnea, restless leg syndrome, periodic limb movement disorder, REM-behavior disorder
- Multiple sleep latency test to assess degree of sleepiness
- Testing for underlying conditions as necessary (e.g., TSH, ECG, chest X-ray, EEG, iron studies, LFTs, tox screen)

Treatment/Management

- Acute transient insomnia: Reassurance, address stressors, treat identifiable underlying causes (e.g., pain), hypnotic agents for up to 7–10 d
- Chronic insomnia
  - Improve sleep hygiene (e.g., consistent bed/wake time, sleep environment, medications/drugs, limit daytime naps, hot bath near bedtime)
  - Treat pain and underlying medical/psych issues
  - Behavioral treatments: Relaxation therapy, sleep restriction therapy (curtail time in bed to improve sleep efficiency), stimulus control therapy (bed only for sleep), cognitive therapy (restructure negative thoughts about sleep/daytime functioning)
  - Medications are often used (e.g., benzodiazepines) but there is no proof of long-term efficacy or safety
- Obstructive sleep apnea: Weight loss, CPAP, surgery
- Restless leg syndrome: Dopaminergic agents (e.g., carbidopa/levodopa), benzodiazepines, or opiates

Prognosis/Complications

- Prognosis is usually good if patient is cooperative with the therapeutic regimen

135. Narcolepsy

Etiology/Pathophysiology

- The irresistible urge to fall asleep
- Occurs several times a day, particularly after meals or in boring circumstances
- Usually begins in the second or third decades of life
- May be associated with cataplexy (loss of tone in extremities during laughter or emotional excess), hypnagogic hallucinations, and sleep paralysis
- Family history is frequently present
    - HLA DQBI*0602 gene locus is associated in 90% of cases of narcolepsy and cataplexy
- May be related to a loss of hypocretin/orexin secreting neurons in hypothalamus
- May be associated with CNS diseases (e.g., multiple sclerosis, trauma, brain tumors)—"symptomatic narcolepsy"

Differential Dx

- Obstructive sleep apnea
- Pickwickian syndrome
- Kleine-Levin syndrome
- Insomnia
- Psychiatric disturbance
- Idiopathic hypersomnolence (likely forme fruste) of narcolepsy
- Drug seeking

Presentation/Signs & Symptoms

- Hypersomnolence
- Cataplexy: Loss of muscle tone during wakefulness or at times of strong emotion
- Hypnagogic hallucinations: Vivid dreams, at times difficult to separate from reality
- Sleep paralysis: Inability to move when awake—occurs at sleep onset in narcolepsy

Diagnostic Evaluation

- History and physical examination
- Multiple sleep latency tests
    - Average sleep onset for four daytime naps less than 10 min, usually less than 5 min
    - At least two naps with REM onset in first 20 min of sleep
- Rapid induction of REM sleep on EEG

Treatment/Management

- Treatment is generally lifelong
- Frequent naps may be beneficial
- Stimulants (e.g., pemoline, modafinil, methylphenidate, methamphetamine)
- γ-Hydroxybutyrate is used and may also improve cataplexy, sleep paralysis, and hypnagogic hallucinations
- Cataplexy particularly difficult to treat; imipramine is often used

Prognosis/Complications

- Complications of daytime hypersomnolence, including inability to drive
- Medication side effects include hypertension, insomnia, irritability, and drug dependence
- May limit the ability to participate in jobs that require alertness (e.g., operating heavy equipment, piloting, driving, soldiering)

136. Obstructive Sleep Apnea

Etiology/Pathophysiology

- Sleep apnea syndrome is a clinical definition that includes the presence of episodes of apnea, hypopnea, and symptoms of functional impairment; results in frequent oxygen desaturations and marked fragmentation of sleep, causing daytime symptoms
- May be obstructive, central, or mixed (symptoms are similar regardless)
    - Obstructive: Upper airway soft tissue impedes airflow; risk factors include narrow airways (obesity, macroglossia), alcohol, sedatives, URI, hypothyroidism, smoking, vocal cord dysfunction, bulbar disease
    - Central: Absent signal to breathe from the CNS respiratory center; apnea without respiratory effort; may be caused by medications (e.g., narcotics, benzodiazepines, alcohol); also seen in brainstem dysfunction, head injury, and CHF
- Occurs in 2% of women and 4% of men
- Most common in obese, middle-aged men
- Obstructive apnea more common than central apnea
- Central apnea is more common at the extremes of age
- There is often snoring for many years prior to the onset of actual obstruction; thus, snoring alone is not a reason for full workup

Differential Dx

- Narcolepsy
- Idiopathic hypersomnolence
- Insomnia
- Primary alveolar hypoventilation ("Ondine's curse"): inadequate ventilation with hypoxemia despite normal airflow, normal pulmonary system and normal respiratory drive
- Pickwickian syndrome: Hypoventilation due to blunted central drive plus increased mechanical load of the chest wall
- Hypothyroidism

Presentation/Signs & Symptoms

- Sleep apnea syndrome is one of the leading causes of daytime sleepiness
- Loud snoring
- Restlessness/thrashing during sleep
- Breath cessations or respiratory efforts without air flow while sleeping
- Obesity
- Narrowed oropharynx
- Daytime somnolence and fatigue
- Morning sluggishness
- Cognitive impairment
- Headaches
- Impotence
- Personality changes
- The patient's bed partner often provides the most useful information

Diagnostic Evaluation

- History and physical examination: Workup is appropriate when nocturnal problems are contributing to secondary daytime behavioral and physiologic problems
- Initial laboratory testing may include CBC (may show erythrocytosis) and thyroid function studies
- Overnight pulse oximetry is a useful screening test
    - Highly sensitive and sufficient to establish the diagnosis in patients with a high pretest probability of the disease
    - If normal, it excludes the diagnosis in patients with a low pretest probability of the disease
- Overnight polysomnography is diagnostic
    - Monitors physiology during sleep, including EEG, EMG, ECG, oximetry, airflow, and respiratory effort
    - Shows apneic episodes and provides a definitive diagnosis
    - A positive test has 10 apneic or hypopneic episodes per h lasting at least 10 s each
    - Lack of respiratory effort occurs in central apnea

Treatment/Management

- Patients with increased upper airway muscle tone should avoid alcohol and sedatives
- For patients with decreased upper airway lumen size:
    - Weight reduction may be curative
    - Oral dental prosthesis
    - Nasal septoplasty if deviated septum is present
    - Uvulopalatopharyngoplasty in selected patients
- Nighttime nasal CPAP is treatment of choice; 100% effective but may be very uncomfortable
- Bypass occlusion (e.g., tracheostomy) may be necessary in patients with life-threatening complications and failure of other therapies
- Oxygen may worsen apnea and should be prescribed only after observing patient with polysomnography
- Central sleep apnea is difficult to treat due to CNS dysfunction; tricyclic antidepressants may decrease episodes, thereby improving daytime symptoms

Prognosis/Complications

- Sleep apnea does cause increased mortality
- Repetitive hypoxia may ultimately result in cardiac arrhythmias, pulmonary hypertension, and cor pulmonale
- Other sequelae include CHF (especially in patients with preexisting left ventricular dysfunction), systemic hypertension, and erythrocytosis
- The disease usually follows a chronic, progressive course due to continued weight gain
- There is a good response to therapy, especially nasal CPAP, but tolerability varies

137. Night Terrors

Etiology/Pathophysiology

- A condition of waking from sleep with extreme agitation, tachycardia, and tachypnea
- Occurs primarily in childhood
- Frequently associated with sleepwalking and enuresis
- Associated with psychiatric disorders (anxiety, stress, personality disorders)
- Occurs in sleep stages 3–4, usually (75% of cases) in the first delta cycle of the night, 60–90 min after sleep onset
- Patients are frequently amnestic of the event

Differential Dx

- Nightmares (occur in REM sleep)
- Nocturnal seizures
- Medications (β-blockers, dopaminergic agents)

Presentation/Signs & Symptoms

- Extreme fright and confusion upon awakening
- Screaming often occurs
- Autonomic phenomenon are present (e.g., tachycardia, tachypnea, diaphoresis, dilated pupils, enuresis)
- Slow recovery upon awakening (10–30 min)
- May be associated with somnambulism (sleepwalking)

Diagnostic Evaluation

- History alone is usually sufficient
- Sleep study or video/EEG monitoring may be necessary

Treatment/Management

- Benzodiazepines and SSRIs may be useful by decreasing sleep stages 3 and 4 and as an anxiolytic
- Psychotherapy may be indicated

Prognosis/Complications

- Usually self-limited
- Frequently disappears by adulthood
- Response to treatment is variable

Miscellaneous Neurologic Conditions

JON BRILLMAN, MD, FRCPI
THOMAS F. SCOTT, MD

138. Subdural Hematoma

Etiology/Pathophysiology

- Acute subdural hematoma occurs in association with severe closed head injury
  - The most common and most lethal of posttraumatic intracranial lesions
  - Typically due to shearing of cortical veins with significant associated brain injury
  - Commonly associated with parenchymal brain lesions, such as contusions, hematoma, and diffuse axonal injury
  - Increased frequency in the elderly, especially those on anticoagulation (in the elderly, the trauma may seem trivial or not even noted)
- Chronic subdural hematoma presents 1–2 mo after a usually trivial, and often unremembered, head trauma
  - Initially, small amounts of subdural blood collect
  - Progressive enlargement occurs due to defects in local fibrinolytic pathways or anticoagulation
- Secondary brain injury: Additional insults following injury (e.g., hypotension, hypoxia, brain swelling) may propagate further cerebral tissue damage by decreasing cerebral perfusion pressure
- Alcoholics are prone to subdurals because of trauma and coagulopathies

Differential Dx

- Acute subdural hematoma
  - Intracranial mass lesion (e.g., epidural hematoma, intracerebral hematoma, abscess)
  - Spontaneous intracerebral hematoma (e.g., hypertensive)
  - Seizure disorder
  - Drug intoxication
  - Metabolic coma
- Chronic subdural
  - Dementia
  - Intracranial mass lesion
  - Seizure disorder
  - Drug intoxication
  - Metabolic disturbances
  - Tension headache
  - Subdural hygroma

Presentation/Signs & Symptoms

- Acute subdural hematoma
  - Patient typically presents in a coma soon after trauma
  - Progressive deterioration and deepening coma, often with decerebrate posturing
  - Focal neurologic signs
- Chronic subdural hematoma
  - Slowly developing symptoms with gradual neurologic symptoms
  - Headaches
  - Progressive drowsiness
  - Mental status changes
  - Gait disturbance
  - Seizures
  - Focal neurologic signs
- Dilated, light-fixed pupil on side of lesion if herniation occurs

Diagnostic Evaluation

- History and physical exam, including a detailed neurologic examination
- Head CT without contrast will show a crescent-shaped, concave hyperdensity (in acute subdural) or hypodensity (in chronic subdural), cerebral edema, and mass effect with shift of midline structures
  - Contrast enhancement helps outline membranes
- Head MRI is indicated if chronic subdural hematoma is suspected to distinguish from a hygroma (benign CSF collection)
- EEG and CSF exams are not recommended for diagnostic purposes

Treatment/Management

- Airway, breathing, and circulation
- Seizure prophylaxis (e.g., phenytoin)
- Acute subdural hematoma
  - Surgical evacuation and control of bleeding if patient is neurologically salvageable
  - ICP monitoring and treatment
  - Prevent/ameliorate secondary brain injuries (IV fluid to prevent hypotension; intubation to prevent hypoxia; and relieve increased ICP by head elevation, mild hyperventilation, mannitol and/or furosemide administration, surgical drainage)
- Chronic subdural hematoma
  - If significant signs are not present, patients may be managed conservatively with monitoring of neurologic status and serial CT scans
  - Evacuation of hematoma with or without associated drainage of subdural space

Prognosis/Complications

- Acute subdural hematoma has a very poor prognosis
  - >80% mortality, usually due to underlying brain injury
  - Early surgical intervention (<4 h from time of injury) may slightly improve outcome
  - Complications are usually related to the need for prolonged ventilation (e.g., pneumonia, ARDS, sepsis, multisystem organ failure)
- Chronic subdural hematoma generally has a good prognosis as long as significant focal neurologic signs or coma are not present
  - >80% of cases have a satisfactory outcome
  - The hematoma may reaccumulate or recur, requiring additional surgical interventions
- Elderly patients are often slow to recover
- Recurrence may occur in 20% of cases

139. Epidural Hematoma

Etiology/Pathophysiology

- An uncommon result of closed head injuries; usually associated with a skull fracture
- Most common in 15–30-y-old males following a motor vehicle crash; seen also after falls or sporting activities
- Epidural bleeding most often occurs in the frontotemporal regions secondary to damage of the middle meningeal artery or its branches, resulting in rapid neurologic signs and symptoms
  - Arterial bleeding leads to a rapid rise in ICP, followed by uncal herniation and brainstem compression
- Venous bleeding may occur secondary to venous sinus injuries or "venous lakes" in the dura, resulting in a relatively slow onset of neurologic signs/symptoms; common in the posterior fossa in children
- Secondary brain injury: Additional insults following injury (e.g., hypotension, hypoxia, brain swelling) may propagate further cerebral tissue damage by decreasing cerebral perfusion pressure

Differential Dx

- Intracranial mass lesion
  - Subdural hematoma
  - Intracerebral hematoma
  - Contusion
  - Tumor
- Seizure disorder
- Drug intoxication
- Metabolic coma
- Stroke
- Traumatic subarachnoid hemorrhage

Presentation/Signs & Symptoms

- History of head injury followed by a lucid interval (up to 60 min) and subsequent neurologic decline to coma
- Severe headache
- Seizures
- Vomiting (especially in children)
- Brainstem herniation is indicated by palsy of the third cranial nerve, usually resulting in ipsilateral pupil dilation, and contralateral hemiparesis
- "Cushing effect" is common in children due to pressure on the medulla: Bradycardia, bradypnea, and hypertension

Diagnostic Evaluation

- History and physical exam, including detailed neurologic exam
- Emergent head CT or MRI without contrast: Findings include convex hyperdensity, shift of midline structures, compression of ipsilateral ventricles, and dilation of contralateral ventricles
- C-spine films may be indicated to rule out associated cervical injury
- Lumbar puncture is contraindicated

Treatment/Management

- Attention to airway, breathing, and circulation
- Seizure prophylaxis in all patients (e.g., phenytoin)
- Surgical evacuation with control of bleeding source
- Begin ICP monitoring (i.e., via ventricular catheter or fiber optic monitor) if consciousness is not rapidly regained
- Prevent/ameliorate secondary brain injury
  - IV fluid administration to prevent hypotension
  - Intubation for hypoxia
  - Mannitol or furosemide administration to relieve cerebral edema
  - Relieve elevated ICP by head elevation, mild hyperventilation (e.g., $pCO_2 = 35$), mannitol and/or furosemide administration, and surgical drainage
- Burr-hole evacuation if no other treatment is available

Prognosis/Complications

- Excellent outcome if treated early
- Rarely associated with other significant intracranial injuries
- 20% mortality
- Sudden death may occur
- If patient is comatose and decerebrate, prognosis is grim as a brainstem compression has occurred as a result of transtentorial herniation of temporal lobe

MISCELLANEOUS NEUROLOGIC CONDITIONS

140. Bell's Palsy

Etiology/Pathophysiology

- A sudden weakness of the face involving the distribution of CN VII to the muscles of facial expression
- Pathophysiology involves edema of the facial nerve, which likely becomes compressed in the facial canal or foramen spinosum
- A common disorder that affects men and women equally at all ages
- The most common cause of facial nerve paralysis
- Often follows exposure to cold or wind for unclear reasons
- There is some association with elevated herpes-1 titers
- Bell's palsy is a peripheral or lower motor neuron palsy; differentiate supranuclear facial palsy from peripheral (nuclear) facial palsy
  - Supranuclear palsy predominantly involves the lower part of the face; emotional responses may be intact (e.g., the patient may not be able to show you his teeth but will smile in response to a joke)
  - Peripheral, or nuclear facial palsy, affects all ipsilateral muscles of facial expression, resulting in paralysis of the entire ipsilateral side; the angle of mouth is pulled to the normal side and may droop on the affected side, facial creases are effaced, and the affected eyelid may not close

Differential Dx

- Stroke (Bell's palsy involves the entire face with inability to close eye completely, whereas strokes affect the lower part of the face primarily)
- Hemifacial spasm
- Lyme disease
- Guillain-Barré syndrome
- Acoustic neuroma
- Herpes zoster (Ramsay Hunt syndrome)
- Ectatic basilar artery and compression of facial nerve
- Hysterical facial contractures, including blepharospasm
- Multiple sclerosis

Presentation/Signs & Symptoms

- Paresis or paralysis of facial muscles, including eye closure, reaches maximum weakness within 48 h
- Retroauricular pain often precedes the paralysis
- Occasional tingling sensation of face
- Ipsilateral loss of taste due to involvement of chordae tympani
- Ipsilateral hyperacusis due to involvement of stapedius muscle
- Ipsilateral "crocodile" tears may develop due to aberrant attempt at reinnervation
- Bell's phenomenon (upward deviation of eye with attempted eye closure)
- Drooling of mouth at side of paresis
- Irritation of cornea may occur secondary to impaired eye closure

Diagnostic Evaluation

- Neuroimaging may be obtained to exclude posterior fossa lesions if presentation is atypical or concerning
- EMG and nerve conduction studies of the facial nerve; if denervation is present after 2 wk, prognosis for recovery may be prolonged
- Lumbar puncture is not necessary unless Lyme disease or GBS is suspected
- Lyme antibody titer is only indicated if other clinical features of Lyme disease are present (e.g., arthralgias, characteristic rash)

Treatment/Management

- A tapered course of prednisone will relieve the retroauricular pain but it is uncertain if it helps the facial palsy
- Eye protection is necessary, including eye occluder at night and eye drops
- Gentle massage of the face is recommended
- Electrical stimulation has not been shown to be of benefit
- Surgical decompression is not beneficial and not recommended

Prognosis/Complications

- 80% of cases recover within 2–3 wk
- 10% of cases may take up to a year to recover
- 10% of cases do not recover and develop synkenesis of face (contracture of muscles)
- Ability to close eye is favorable prognostic sign
- Recovery of taste is a favorable prognostic sign
- Diabetics and hypertensive patients may have a worse prognosis for full recovery

141. Hemifacial Spasm

Etiology/Pathophysiology

- A painless, irregular contraction of the facial muscles on one side of the face
- Most cases are due to demyelination or facial nerve root compression by an artery or vein
- Injured fibers become irritable and cause continual contraction of the muscles of facial expression
- Often a sequela of Bell's palsy
- Generally begins in fifth or sixth decade of life

Differential Dx

- Bell's palsy
- Tic or habit spasm
- Tourette's syndrome
- Fatigue-induced fasciculations of orbicularis oculi
- Partial seizure
- Facial myokymia
- Blepharospasm

Presentation/Signs & Symptoms

- Continual contractions of facial muscles on one side of face
- Mild facial muscle weakness
- Contractions are often induced by facial movements

Diagnostic Evaluation

- Magnification MRI or MRA of the posterior fossa and posterior circulation may indicate compression of the facial nerve by a vascular structure

Treatment/Management

- Tegretol will control spasms in half of cases
- Gabapentin or baclofen may be helpful
- Botox injections into facial muscles
- Posterior fossa microvascular decompression if necessary is beneficial in 90% of cases

Prognosis/Complications

- Recurrence in 10–20% of cases

142. Transient Global Amnesia

Etiology/Pathophysiology

- A brief syndrome of amnesia seen in migraine patients and elderly patients
- Transient dysfunction of memory, both retrograde and anterograde, with intact cognition
- Etiology is uncertain; likely secondary to ischemia to the medial temporal lobes
- May be precipitated by emotional events
- Coronary and cerebral angiography may cause vasospasm resulting in ischemia and amnesia
- Has also been reported after sexual intercourse and sedative hypnotics

Differential Dx

- Complex partial seizure
- Nonconvulsive status epilepsy
- Transient ischemic attack
- Hypoglycemia
- Drug or alcohol intoxication
- Posttraumatic amnesia
- Psychogenic fugue state (hysterical amnesia)
- Postictal state

Presentation/Signs & Symptoms

- Mild headache
- Retrograde and anterograde amnesia lasting several hours
- The patient is alert and interactive with the environment but asks repeated questions about where they are and why they are there
- Patient is able to carry on some activities but seems bewildered
- After episode is over, memory is lost for that period of time
- No loss of memory for self

Diagnostic Evaluation

- Head CT or MRI to rule out stroke or structural lesion
- EEG to exclude seizure activity
- MRA may be indicated to evaluate the vertebrobasilar circulation, which supplies the functional regions of the temporal lobe

Treatment/Management

- No specific treatment is recommended
- Patients are often placed on aspirin or migraine prophylaxis if associated with migraine

Prognosis/Complications

- Prognosis is good
- Recurrence rate is low, in range of 5%
- Does not appear to be a risk factor for stroke

143. Congenital Neurologic Malformations

Etiology/Pathophysiology

- Arnold-Chiari malformation is a posterior fossa abnormality of two major types
    - Type I is most common: The cerebellar tonsils project 4 mm below the foramen magnum into the cervical area; many are asymptomatic and detected incidentally on MRI
    - Type II malformations include the downward projection of the cerebellar tonsils and displacement of the medulla, and are associated with hydrocephalus and meningomyelocele in the lumbar area
    - Hydrocephalus and syringomyelia is common in both types (50% of cases): These are cystic cavities in the center of the spinal cord, usually in the cervical region, which cause spasticity in legs and arms, hypalgesia across shoulders (cape distribution), amyotrophy of hands, and loss of pain sensation in hands and arms with retention of light touch and vibratory sensation
- Dandy-Walker syndrome is an agenesis of the midline of the cerebellum with large posterior fossa cyst; upper displacement of the tentorium occurs
- Hydrocephalus may lead to mental retardation

Differential Dx

- Cerebral palsy
- Multiple sclerosis
- Cerebellar degeneration
- Cervical myelopathies
- Tumors of foramen magnum
- Congenital hydrocephalus
- Platybasia or basilar impression

Presentation/Signs & Symptoms

- Type I: Often asymptomatic but later in life may be associated with hydrocephalus and headache, downbeat nystagmus, lower cranial nerve abnormalities, and spastic quadraparesis
- Type II is associated with hydrocephalus and meningomyelocele in childhood with multiple cranial neuropathies
- Meningomyelocele is manifested by flaccid paralysis of legs, dribbling of urine, absent reflexes, loss of sensation in legs and sacral areas; meningitis is common due to exposure of lumbar root and meninges to external environment
- Mental retardation common with Dandy-Walker syndrome
- Seizures

Diagnostic Evaluation

- MRI of brain with sagittal views will identify all cases
- Cervical MRI if syringomyelia or hydromyelia is suspected
- Lumbar MRI will detect meningomyeloceles

Treatment/Management

- Ventriculoatrial or ventriculoperitoneal shunting may be necessary for hydrocephalus
- Chiari malformations may require posterior fossa decompression
    - If associated with hydromyelia, enlargement of the posterior fossa and decompression of cervical region is necessary; drainage of hydromyelia has variable results
- Surgical intervention and covering of meningomyelocele may prevent meningitis
- Anticonvulsant medication may be necessary

Prognosis/Complications

- Type I malformations have favorable prognosis unless syringomyelia is present or surgical intervention is necessary
- Type II malformations have a poor prognosis; few patients survive to adulthood
- Hydromyelia or syringomyelia have poor prognosis in terms of function; patients are frequently wheelchair-bound
- Dandy-Walker syndrome and meningomyelocele have poor prognoses; patients rarely survive to adulthood
- Mental retardation and seizures are common
- Recurrent meningitis is common with meningomyeloceles

144. Neurofibromatosis

Etiology/Pathophysiology

- These are common disorders with autosomal-dominant inheritance that result in abnormalities in skin, bones, and the nervous system associated with multiple benign tumors
- Neurofibromas are benign tumors of Schwann cells; they may be felt as nodules along peripheral nerves
- There are two distinct disorders with separate gene abnormalities
- NF-1 (von Recklinghausen's disease) is one of the most common genetic disorders (30–40 per 100,000)
    - Associated with skin lesions and subcutaneous and peripheral nerve lesions as well as plexiform neuromas, osseous abnormalities (portions of facial bones may be absent), and gliomas (often of the optic nerves)
- NF-2 is less common and does not include involvement of other organ systems
    - Associated with bilateral acoustic neuromas
    - Presents in young adulthood

Differential Dx

- Tuberous sclerosis
- Meningiomas
- Schwannoma of acoustic nerve
- Benign hamartomas
- Astrocytoma

Presentation/Signs & Symptoms

- NF-1: Café au lait spots; axillary and inguinal freckles; Lisch nodules on iris; plexiform neuromas (large subcutanous masses on face); cutaneous and subcutaneous tumors on trunk, abdomen, and extremities; optic gliomas; bony cysts; pathologic fractures; obstructive hydrocephalus; spinal root tumors; seizures; pheochromocytoma may be present; intellectual impairment in 40% of cases
- NF-2: Hearing loss, tinnitus, vertigo, facial pain, gait ataxia and imbalance, absence of corneal reflex, headache

Diagnostic Evaluation

- Diagnosis of NF-1 requires two or more of: First-degree relative with NF-1; bone lesions; axillary/inguinal freckles; two neurofibromas; Lisch nodules, optic gliomas; and/or five or more café au lait spots
- Diagnosis of NF-2 requires one of the following: Bilateral acoustic neuromas (CN VIII tumor) on MRI; first-degree relative with NF-2 and a unilateral acoustic neuroma or two other associated tumors
- Biopsy of subcutaneous nodules may be useful
- MRI with contrast of brain and spine to evaluate for spinal tumors
- EEG may be necessary to evaluate for seizure activity
- 24-h urine for epinephrine metabolites if suspect pheochromocytoma
- Brainstem auditory evoked responses
- Audiograms to evaluate for hearing loss

Treatment/Management

- No cure exists; treatment is based on managing symptoms and associated tumors
- NF-1
    - Surgery for accessible tumors
    - Treatment and prevention of seizures
    - Orthopedic procedures for orthopedic deformities
    - Ophthalmologic surveillance and/or radiation therapy for optic gliomas
- NF-2
    - Yearly auditory evaluation
    - Surgical debulking of acoustic neuromas
    - Screening for associated CNS tumors with periodic brain imaging
- Anticonvulsants for seizures
- Shunting for hydrocephalus
- Plastic surgery intervention may be appropriate
- Genetic counseling

Prognosis/Complications

- NF-1 may have aggressive course with increased risk of brain tumors, Wilms' tumor, neuroblastoma
- Families with NF should undergo genetic counseling, as there is no cure for the disease
- Disease is progressive but may remain mild with few cutaneous and subcutaneous lesions
- May be severe with mental retardation, seizures, severe physical deformities, and neoplasms

145. Tuberous Sclerosis

Etiology/Pathophysiology

- A congenital neurocutaneous syndrome resulting in childhood seizures and variable mental retardation
- Autosomal dominant inheritance
- The abnormal genes have been localized to long arm of chromosome 9 and short arm of 16
- Tumors of the brain and other organs are prominent
- As with neurofibromatosis, the clinical expression is extremely variable, although most affected patients have seizures

Differential Dx

- Neurofibromatosis
- Albright's syndrome
- Posterior fossa tumors
- Astrocytoma
- Metastatic brain cancer
- Cerebral palsy
- Von Hippel-Lindau disease
- Epilepsy

Presentation/Signs & Symptoms

- Infancy: Infantile spasms
- Childhood: Seizures, ash leaf spots, Shagreen patches, retinal hamartomas, renal angiolipomas, cardiac rhabdomyosarcomas, periungual fibromas, CNS tumors, subependymal nodules, and astrocytomas
- Skin lesions include hypomelanotic macules or reverse café au lait spots on trunk or limbs
- Seizures occur in 75% of cases beginning in the first year of life and often manifest as mixed patterns or infantile spasms
- Progressive mental retardation is variable
- Choreic movements
- Quadrispasticity

Diagnostic Evaluation

- Classic triad of epilepsy, mental retardation, and adenoma sebaceum (subcutaneous tumors in region of sebaceous glands)
- Other typical skin, retinal, and brain lesions are present
- CNS tumors and cardiac rhabdomyomas may be seen on prenatal ultrasound
- EEG may show hypsarrhythmia
- CT or MRI of brain to demonstrate ventricular surface lesions, described as "candle drippings"

Treatment/Management

- No cures exist; treatment is based on managing symptoms and associated tumors
- Treatment and prevention of seizures, including surgical removal of epileptogenic tumors
- Infantile spasms are often treated successfully with ACTH
- Renal and cardiac monitoring for associated tumors
- Genetic counseling
- Surgical excision of tumors is rarely indicated

Prognosis/Complications

- Patients may have refractory epilepsy and renal complications; cardiac lesions usually recede after the newborn period
- Psychiatric problems (e.g., autism)
- The younger the presentation, the worse the prognosis
- The primary prognostic indicators of neurocutaneous lesions are the presence of associated neoplasms
- Patients are often mentally handicapped and require special education or speech therapy
- Slow but definite progression
- 50% die before age 50
- Seizures very difficult to control and often lead to status epilepticus
- Tumors of brain often enlarge and become malignant or cause hydrocephalus

146. Metabolic Encephalopathies

Etiology/Pathophysiology

- Altered cerebral function secondary to endogenous toxin buildup as a result of organ failure, including the heart and lungs, kidneys, endocrine organs, liver, and electrolyte balance
- Etiologies include cardiac and respiratory arrest with hypoxia and hypercapnea, diabetes mellitus, hypoglycemia, uremic encephalopathy, dialysis dysequilibrium syndrome and dialysis dementia, hepatic coma, Reye's syndrome, hyperosmolar syndrome, hyponatremia, metabolic acidosis or alkalosis, hypothyroidism, hypoparathyroidism, dehydration, hypercalcemia, hypocalcemia, and carbon monoxide poisoning

Differential Dx

- Stroke (especially brainstem infarct)
- Wernicke's encephalopathy
- Brain death
- Intoxications
- Vitamin B_{12} deficiency
- Nonconvulsive status or postictal state
- Cerebral neoplasm
- Central pontine myelinolysis
- Wilson's disease
- Posttraumatic encephalopathy
- Cerebral hemorrhage
- Subarachnoid hemorrhage
- Meningitis
- Dementia
- Transient global amnesia

Presentation/Signs & Symptoms

- Delirium
- Confusion
- Drowsiness possibly progressing to stupor and coma
- Asterixis
- Multifocal myoclonus
- Small, reactive pupils
- Seizures
- Headache
- Nausea and vomiting
- Decorticate and decerebrate posturing
- Cheyne-Stokes respirations
- Extrapyramidal signs
- Babinski sign
- Tetany (hypocalcemia and alkalosis)

Diagnostic Evaluation

- Initial laboratory tests may include chemistries, renal function tests, LFTs, CBC, calcium level, thyroid function tests, drug screen, ammonia level, serum osmolarity, and arterial blood gas
- Brain imaging with CT scan or MRI
- EEG shows slowing and frequently triphasic waves

Treatment/Management

- Attention to airway, breathing, and circulation
- Intubation may be necessary
- Rehydration as necessary
- Seizures should be treated with IV phenytoin
- Correct metabolic abnormalities as rapidly as possible, except for hyponatremia which should be corrected slowly to avoid central pontine myelinolysis
- Dialysis may be necessary for renal failure with uremia
- Lactulose and neomycin enemas for hepatic encephalopathy
- Insulin for diabetic coma
- Glucose for hypoglycemia
- Calcium gluconate for hypocalcemia

Prognosis/Complications

- Prognosis depends on the specific metabolic abnormality and rate of correction
- In general, hypoxia and uremia have the worst prognoses, especially if seizures are present

147. Swallowing Disturbances

Etiology/Pathophysiology

- Swallowing is a complex neurologic function requiring the integration of several regions of the nervous system
- Patients with neurologic swallowing difficulties generally have more problems with liquids than solids
- Normally, unilateral cerebral damage does not produce dysphagia, although frontal or parietal lesions may cause apraxia of swallowing
- Bilateral cortical or subcortical lesions may cause pseudobulbar palsy with an exaggerated gag reflex and spasm of the cricopharyngeal muscle
- Patients with Parkinson's disease or progressive supranuclear palsy with extrapyramidal disorders may have rigidity of muscles of deglutition
- Patients with brainstem lesions (e.g., lateral medullary stroke, or Wallenberg's syndrome) frequently have swallowing disturbances that slowly improve with time
- ALS and other disorders of cranial nerve nuclei (e.g., polio) adversely affect swallowing
- Neuropathies including diphtheria and GBS often cause dysphagia
- Disorders of neuromuscular junction (myasthenia gravis) cause dysphagia
- Polymyositis and rare forms of muscular dystrophy affect swallowing

Differential Dx

- Strokes in the cerebral hemispheres
- Alzheimer's disease
- Binswanger's disease
- CJD
- Parkinson's disease
- Progressive supranuclear palsy
- Shy-Drager syndrome
- Brainstem strokes
- GBS
- Diphtheria
- ALS
- Polio
- Myasthenia gravis
- Botulism
- Polymyositis
- Skull base metastasis
- Meningeal carcinomatosis

Presentation/Signs & Symptoms

- Difficulty initiating swallowing with buildup of food in oropharynx
- Nasal regurgitation of liquids
- Choking and coughing
- Hyperactive or hypoactive gag reflex
- Absence of gag reflex unilaterally
- Aspiration, sometimes silent
- Drooling
- Paresis of lingual movements
- Nasal speech

Diagnostic Evaluation

- Clinical observation of swallowing may reveal regurgitation, particularly of liquids through the nose, or signs of aspiration
- 30 cc water swallow test at bedside to evaluate swallowing
- Videofluoroscopy (modified barium swallow) will identify aspiration and buildup of food in the oropharynx
- Chest X-ray if suspect aspiration pneumonia

Treatment/Management

- Speech therapy consult
- Dysphagia diets (soft, mechanical diets that are easy to swallow with minimal chewing)
- Drink through straw (smaller amounts may be negotiable)
- Feeding tubes (J or G tube) may be necessary until swallowing function returns
- Flexiflow nasogastric tubes
- Cricopharyngeal myotomy may help in pseudobulbar palsy

Prognosis/Complications

- Prognosis depends entirely on the etiology of dysphagia
- With care to prevent aspiration, most cases with cerebral or brainstem infarction will improve

148. Posterior Reversible Encephalopathy Syndrome

Etiology/Pathophysiology

- A condition of cerebral edema resulting from dysautoregulation of the cerebral circulation
  - Normally, cerebral autoregulation ensures that cerebral blood flow remains relatively constant despite large fluctuations in blood pressure
- Commonly seen with severe hypertension, eclampsia of pregnancy, and use of chemotherapeutic agents (e.g., cyclosporine)
- Edema occurs in the white matter primarily by gray matter may be involved
- Edema is usually in the posterior portions of brain but may be anywhere
- Cerebellum and brainstem may be involved

Differential Dx

- TIA
- Strokes, especially top of the basilar syndrome
- Reye's syndrome
- Call's syndrome (vasculopathy of puerperium)
- Cortical vein thrombosis
- Cerebral tumors with
- Hemolytic-uremic syndrome
- Thrombotic-thrombocy-topenic purpura

Presentation/Signs & Symptoms

- Confusion
- Headache
- Seizures
- Visual blurring
- Nausea and vomiting
- Focal neurologic findings

Diagnostic Evaluation

- MRI demonstrates edema of white matter often extending into the gray matter
  - Microinfarcts and hemorrhages may be seen

Treatment/Management

- Treatment involves reversal of the underlying cause
  - Hypertensive crisis should be treated with nitroprusside
  - Magnesium sulfate for eclampsia
  - Discontinuation of chemotherapeutic agents
- Nimodipine may be helpful

Prognosis/Complications

- Prognosis is generally favorable if hypertension can be controlled
- Edema of brain resolves postpartum

149. Fibromyalgia

Etiology/Pathophysiology

- A fairly common syndrome of chronic, generalized muscular pain
- Formerly known as fibrositis; however, this term is a misnomer as there are no signs of inflammation
- Idiopathic; may be related to viral disease, psychiatric factors, sleep disorders, or hypothyroidism
- May be a rheumatologic or autoimmune illness although no specific tissue pathology has been identified
- Widespread muscular involvement with multiple, bilateral, fibromyalgia-specific "tender points"
- Often seen with chronic fatigue complaints and nonspecific complaints such as poor concentration, headaches, paresthesias
- Especially affects women ages 20 to 50
- May affect as much as 10% of the general population

Differential Dx

- Depression
- Chronic fatigue syndrome
- Polymyositis
- Rheumatoid arthritis
- Myofascial pain syndrome
- Polymyalgia rheumatica
- SLE
- Ankylosing spondylitis
- Hypothyroidism
- Viral syndrome
- Lyme disease
- Sjögren's syndrome
- Sarcoidosis
- Multiple sclerosis
- Metabolic disorders (e.g., hypothyroidism, other endocrinopathies)

Presentation/Signs & Symptoms

- Soft tissue pain throughout body, especially back, neck, shoulders, hips
- Gnawing, aching, burning pain
- Stiffness and soreness with inactivity; pain not relieved by rest
- Increased symptoms as day progresses
- Symptoms worsen with stress and tension
- Tenderness out of proportion to palpation
- Bilateral focal tender points
- Fatigue and sleep disturbance common
- Nonspecific symptoms may be present, including abdominal pain, bloating, alternating diarrhea/constipation, susceptibility to cold, numbness, poor concentration, headache, depression
- Normal neurologic exam

Diagnostic Evaluation

- History and physical most important
- Diagnosis of exclusion: Lack of laboratory abnormalities
- 11 of 18 characteristic tender points must be present for diagnosis
- Rule out RA and SLE: Check ESR and ANA titers
- Rule out hypothyroidism: Check thyroid function tests
- Rule out trauma, infection, rheumatic disease
- EMG and EEG may rule out other diseases
- MRI may be indicated if headaches or cognitive complaints coexist

Treatment/Management

- Reassurance and counseling
- Continued monitoring for signs of systemic illness, regular checkups
- Physical therapy or gentle exercise program with concentration on stretching and consideration of massage therapy or chiropractic manipulation
- Stress reduction and relaxation techniques
- Trials of NSAIDs, tricyclic antidepressants, SSRIs, acetaminophen, or tramadol may be useful
- 1% lidocaine injections into tender points in severe pain
- Considerations can be given to trials of anticonvulsants (e.g., neurontin)
- Avoid opioids and steroids

Prognosis/Complications

- The disease follows a chronic course that can be improved by judicious exercise, stress reduction, and possibly pharmacologic agents
- Patients should be aware that symptoms of fibromyalgia tend to wax and wane over months and years, often impacted by other health issues, social stressors, level of depression, and activity level

150. Traumatic Brain Injury

Etiology/Pathophysiology

- Brain injury is a significant cause of morbidity/mortality in trauma patients
- Patients present along a spectrum from normal physical exam with minimal underlying cognitive dysfunction to a vegetative state
- Leading cause of death in persons under the age of 50
- Primary injury occurs at the time of trauma
- Secondary injury occurs after the initial insult due to hypoperfusion (i.e., hypotension, increased ICP), hypoxia, hyperglycemia, or anemia
- Intracranial hemorrhage can occur into the epidural space, subdural space (acute or chronic), subarachnoid space, or intraparenchymal tissue
- Penetrating injury (usually gunshot wounds) occurs due to the physical path of the bullet plus associated concussive forces
- Concussive injuries involve a blow to the head that imparts a violent motion of the brain striking the skull
- Concussions cause loss of consciousness due to transient dysfunction of the brainstem; may not be associated with structural brain injury
- Skull fractures are not necessary for severe traumatic brain injuries but are indicators that brain damage is likely to be present
- Basal skull fractures are often associated with CSF rhinorrhea, otorrhea, cranial nerve dysfunction, and carotid-cavernous fistulas

Differential Dx

- Drug/alcohol intoxication
- Hypoglycemia
- Seizure disorder
- Postictal state
- Intracerebral hemorrhage
- Brainstem infarct
- Transient global amnesia
- Anoxic encephalopathy
- Hypoglycemia
- Underlying neurologic condition

Presentation/Signs & Symptoms

- May present with headache, loss of consciousness, pupillary response, or other signs of intracranial hemorrhage
  - Unilateral pupil dilation suggests ipsilateral bleed with herniation
  - Bilateral pupil dilation suggests anoxic injury or bilateral herniation
- Battle's sign (mastoid ecchymosis), raccoon eyes (orbital ecchymosis), and CSF rhinorrhea or otorrhea may signify a basilar skull fracture
- Signs of increased ICP include Cushing's reflex (hypertension, bradycardia, and hypopnea), decreasing level of consciousness, dilated pupils, and posturing (decorticate or decerebrate)

Diagnostic Evaluation

- GCS (eye opening, verbal response, motor response): Simple, reproducible measure of mental status (scale 3–15)
  - Provides information on clinical course, prognosis, and treatment decisions (e.g., intubate if GCS <9)
  - GCS ≤8 indicates severe brain injury, 9–11 indicates moderate injury, and 12–15 indicates mild injury
- C-spine X-ray, CT, or MRI to identify cervical fracture
- Head CT should be performed expeditiously in all patients with suspected closed head injury (indicated by loss of consciousness, seizure, vomiting, amnesia, focal neurologic findings, skull fracture, or penetrating head trauma
  - Cerebral contusion: Intraparenchymal hyperdensity
  - Epidural hematoma: Convex hyperdensity
  - Subdural hematoma (acute): Concave hyperdensity
  - Subdural hematoma (chronic): Concave hypodensity
  - Traumatic subarachnoid: Blood in subarachnoid space

Treatment/Management

- Rapid intervention with particular attention to ABCs is necessary to minimize secondary brain injury
- Treat elevated ICP only if symptomatic
  - Sedate patient and elevate head of bed 30°
  - Brief hyperventilation may be performed acutely to cause cerebral vasoconstriction
  - Mannitol for osmotic diuresis and free radical scavenging
  - Surgical decompression of deteriorating patients via trephination (burr hole) or ventriculostomy
- Intracranial bleeds require seizure prophylaxis (e.g., phenytoin) and may require surgical drainage
- Check coagulation studies (PT/PTT/INR) immediately and correct any coagulopathy to minimize intracranial bleeding
- Depressed skull fractures and penetrating trauma may require surgical repair

Prognosis/Complications

- Neurosurgical evaluation is required for any intracranial lesion
- Mortality increases with secondary brain injury
  - One episode of SBP <90 doubles mortality
  - 40% mortality if initial GCS <9
- Concussions may result in a postconcussive syndrome (vague, persistent symptoms such as headache, dizziness, and poor concentration) for weeks to months
- Patients with apparently normal presentation may have underlying cognitive deficits; neuropsychiatric testing is usually recommended
- Posttraumatic epilepsy occurs in 50% of penetrating head injuries and 5% of closed head injuries; incidence increases with prolonged periods of coma; onset is frequently delayed by several months

151. Brain Herniation Syndromes

Etiology/Pathophysiology

- These are often fatal neurologic syndromes that result from compression of vital brain centers due to displaced brain tissue
- Neurologic signs often develop due to pressure on the compressed anatomic structures by the herniated brain
- Transtentorial herniation is a common accompaniment of a hemispheric mass: Uncus of the temporal lobe is forced through the free edge of the tentorium and the midbrain is compressed
- Central herniation: Downward displacement of the thalamus and subthalamic structures compress the midbrain
- Cingulate herniation: Cingulate gyrus squeezes under the falx to the opposite hemisphere
- Herniation of brain tissue through an open skull due to trauma or surgery
- Herniation of the cerebellar tonsil occurs through the foramen magnum, compressing the medullary structures due to masses in the posterior fossa
- Upward herniation due to cerebellar masses may rarely occur secondary to unusual pressure gradients (e.g., decompression of obstructing hydrocephalus); may result in venous infarction
- Spinal herniations may occur if a lumbar puncture is performed in the presence of a compressive lesion of the spinal cord

Differential Dx

- Drug or alcohol intoxication
- Anoxic encephalopathy
- Brainstem stroke
- Tumor
- Postictal state
- Metabolic encephalopathy
- Cerebral hematoma
- Cerebellar hematoma
- Subdural hematoma

Presentation/Signs & Symptoms

- Headache, nausea/vomiting
- Decerebrate posturing
- Drowsiness progressing to stupor/coma
- Transtentorial herniation: Ipsilateral pupillary dilatation, contralateral hemiparesis/plegia, bilateral Babinski
  - If midbrain is compressed against the contralateral tentorial edge, an ipsilateral hemiparesis or plegia ensues
  - Compression of the posterior cerebral artery against the tentorial edge may produce an occipital infarct and contralateral homonymous hemianopsia
- Cingulate herniation: Possible bilateral leg weakness
- Tonsillar herniation: Stiff neck, downbeat nystagmus, respiratory arrest

Diagnostic Evaluation

- Lumbar puncture is contraindicated in suspected herniation syndromes
- CT and MRI of the brain will demonstrate obliteration of the midbrain cisterns in uncal herniation, protrusion of the cerebellar tonsils in tonsillar herniation, or entrapment of the temporal horn in cingulate herniation

Treatment/Management

- Antiedema measures include reverse Trendelenburg positioning, hyperventilation, mannitol administration, and corticosteroids
- Surgical decompression may be necessary emergently

Prognosis/Complications

- Herniation syndromes are often fatal without timely intervention
- Prognosis depends on the underlying cause (e.g., favorable prognosis in subdural or cerebellar hematomas, unfavorable in malignant tumors)

152. Post-CABG Neurologic Complications

Etiology/Pathophysiology

- Post-CABG encephalopathy is a relatively common consequence of prolonged cardiopulmonary bypass procedures
  - Prolonged bypass pump times is generally considered >1 h
  - Encephalopathy is likely caused by multiple air or particulate microemboli secondary to surgical maneuvers or air emboli from the bypass pump
  - Additional risk factors include valve replacement, calcified ascending aorta, postoperative A-fib, intraoperative hypotension, repeat revascularization procedures or grafts on previously stented vessels, old age
  - There is a 5% risk of stroke, likely of embolic etiology from the aorta or heart
- Brachial plexus injury may occur secondary to traction during sternotomy
  - As the sternum is spread apart by large retractors, the brachial plexus is sometimes stretched and injured
- Ulnar neuropathy may occur secondary to prolonged pressure on elbows

Differential Dx

- Stroke
- Postictal state
- Anesthetic complication
- Drug intoxication
- Hypoxic encephalopathy
- Cerebral hemorrhage
- Alzheimer's disease

Presentation/Signs & Symptoms

- Difficulty in extubating encephalopathic patients
- Confusion, agitation, and delirium following the procedure is common
- Seizures may rarely occur
- Stroke occurs in 5%
- Small, reactive pupils
- Babinski signs
- Coma may occur
- Ulnar distribution weakness or numbness and weakness of the hand
- Brachial plexopathies generally result in proximal shoulder weakness and pain
- Phrenic nerve damage may occur, characterized by diaphragmatic paresis

Diagnostic Evaluation

- MRI may show mild brain swelling or stroke
- Transcranial Doppler may detect microembolic signals
- CSF analysis will show elevated protein S100 or neuron-specific enolase (markers for neuronal damage)
- EMG and nerve conduction studies for peripheral traumatic neuropathy or plexopathy

Treatment/Management

- Preventative measures include alternate sites of aortotomy, raising of intraoperative BP, and nonpump procedures
- Treatment is supportive
  - Patients who are agitated or delirious should be sedated
  - Anticoagulation for A-fib

Prognosis/Complications

- Encephalopathy is associated with 15% mortality
- 15–25% have mild permanent cognitive decline
- Neuropathies and plexopathies have variable prognosis but generally improve with time

153. Reye's Syndrome

Etiology/Pathophysiology

- A disorder of cerebral edema that is associated with a nonicteric hepatic encephalopathy
- Follows viral infections, including varicella and influenza
- Occurs primarily in children and adolescents
- Exacerbated by the use of aspirin

Differential Dx

- Bacterial meningitis
- Viral meningitis
- Pseudotumor cerebri
- Cerebral neoplasm with edema
- Metabolic encephalopathy

Presentation/Signs & Symptoms

- Encephalopathy normally preceded by fever and upper respiratory infection or varicella infection
- Protracted vomiting
- Stupor
- Coma
- Seizures
- Decerebrate posturing
- Loss of brainstem reflexes
- Hepatomegaly
- Hyperpyrexia

Diagnostic Evaluation

- MRI or CT of the brain shows signs of herniation, usually of the cerebellar tonsils
- CSF analysis reveals only increased pressure with normal constituents
- Patients tend to become hypoglycemic secondary to hepatic failure
- Abnormal LFTs, including ALT, AST
- Elevated ammonia level and prothrombin time
- EEG shows slowing with triphasic waves

Treatment/Management

- Avoid use of aspirin and other NSAIDs
- Reduce cerebral edema via intubation and hyperventilation (maintain $pCO_2 > 20$ mmHg) and hypertonic solutions
- Temperature control with cooling blanket
- IV glucose to maintain blood sugar between 150–200
- Neomycin enemas and lactulose to reduce blood ammonia
- Monitoring of intracranial pressure

Prognosis/Complications

- Mortality is >60% if blood ammonia levels are over 500 mg/dL and prolonged coma occurs
- Mortality is less than 10% and full recovery is expected if treatment is initiated prior to coma

154. Normal Pressure Hydrocephalus

Etiology/Pathophysiology

- A communicating hydrocephalus that results in dilatation of the cerebral ventricles and a triad of dementia, gait disturbance, and urinary incontinence
- Generally occurs due to prior CNS insults, such as subarachnoid hemorrhage, head trauma, infection (meningitis), tumors, or aqueductal stenosis
  - May be idiopathic in elderly patients
- Pathophysiology involves impaired absorption of spinal fluid through the basal cisterns or basal foramena due to fibrosis or gliosis
- All ventricles are enlarged out of proportion to any cerebral atrophy
- Pressure is likely elevated initially but once ventricles enlarge it equilibrates and becomes "normal"
- Most common in patients older than 60

Differential Dx

- Other causes of dementia (e.g., Alzheimer's, vascular, infectious, or metabolic dementia)
- Parkinson's disease
- Chronic alcohol abuse
- Psychiatric disturbances
- Gait apraxia of old age
- Obstructive hydrocephalus due to mass lesions

Presentation/Signs & Symptoms

- Classic triad of gait disturbance, dementia, and urinary incontinence
  - Gait apraxia is the main sign: Small, uncertain steps with a wide-based, shuffling gait and a tendency to fall
  - Mild subcortical dementia
  - Urinary incontinence or urgency
- Hyperreflexia in lower extremities
- Weakness, malaise, lethargy
- Signs of increased intracranial pressure (e.g., headache, papilledema, alterations of consciousness) are conspicuously absent

Diagnostic Evaluation

- History and neurological exam
  - Patients often have history of a prior CNS insult
- CT scan or MRI of the head shows communicating hydrocephalus with enlargement of all ventricles out of proportion to the degree of cortical atrophy
  - Increased CSF signal is seen in the periventricular areas of white matter due to transependymal movement of CSF
  - Narrowed cerebral sulci
- Lumbar puncture shows normal or high-normal CSF pressure
  - There is a characteristic transient improvement in gait after CSF drainage
  - Clinical improvement following CSF removal may predict those who will benefit from shunting
- Cisternogram with radioisotope may show reversal of flow of CSF and delayed emptying of ventricles

Treatment/Management

- Removal of CSF via lumbar puncture may provide temporary relief
- Ventriculoperitoneal shunting is the treatment of choice
  - Incontinence is the symptom that shows the most improvement following shunting
  - Some patients with other causes of dementia may transiently improve with VP shunting, but these cases will relapse
  - VP shunting is less effective if there has been a long duration of symptoms

Prognosis/Complications

- Gradual onset and progression of symptoms
- Symptoms may be reversible with treatment
- Shunting is beneficial in about 30% of patients, especially those with gait disturbances or rapid dementia
- Shunt complications include seizures, bleeding, or subdural hematoma

155. Hyperosmolar Non-Ketotic Syndrome

Etiology/Pathophysiology

- A condition of stupor, coma, and seizures associated with extreme hyperglycemia and hyperosmolarity with the absence of ketosis
- Neurologic involvement is caused by dehydration of neurons
- Cerebral dehydration occurs as water moves from the intracellular to extracellular compartments secondary to the increased serum osmolarity
- Occurs in adult-onset (noninsulin-dependent) diabetes or insulin-dependent diabetes mellitus
- Often represents the first manifestation of new-onset DM
- Often triggered or exacerbated by systemic infections, renal failure, dialysis, and the use of certain medications, including thiazides, corticosteroids, and immunosuppressive agents

Differential Dx

- Idiopathic epilepsy
- Symptomatic epilepsy
- Postictal state
- Metabolic encephalopathy
- Head trauma
- Transient global amnesia
- Diabetic ketoacidosis
- Dehydration
- Drug overdose
- Brainstem stroke
- Encephalitis
- Hypoglycemia

Presentation/Signs & Symptoms

- Polyuria and polydipsia
- Stupor
- Coma
- Seizures, either generalized or focal
- Epilepsia partialis continua (continuous seizure activity of an extremity)
- Hemiparesis
- Aphasia
- Homonymous hemianopsia
- Myoclonus

Diagnostic Evaluation

- Laboratory studies include serum glucose level, electrolytes, BUN and creatinine, serum and urine osmolarity, and urine studies
  - BUN/creatinine ratio is increased
  - There is elevated glucose in urine with absence of ketones
  - Patients are often hypokalemic
- Diagnosis requires a serum osmolarity greater than 350 mOsm per kg of H_2O, and serum glucose levels of at least 600 mg/dL
- MRI or CT scan of the brain to evaluate for brain edema and rule out other causes of coma
- Chest X-ray to evaluate for pulmonary edema and pneumonia
- EEG may reveal periodic lateralized epileptiform discharges

Treatment/Management

- Reestablish volume with administration of normal saline
  - Replace half of fluid deficit in first 24 h and the remainder over the next few days
- Insulin should be administered in small doses to treat hyperglycemia
- Potassium replacement
- Benzodiazepines or phenytoin for seizures

Prognosis/Complications

- Poor prognosis with 50% mortality rate
- Diabetes should be managed carefully with frequent glucose measurements to prevent future episodes of hyperglycemia
- Treatment with anticonvulsant medication may be required for up to a year

156. Neurologic Conditions in Pregnancy

Etiology/Pathophysiology

- Risk of stroke is greatly increased by hypercoagulable state of pregnancy, especially in migraine patients
- Seizures are more common during pregnancy due to decreased anticonvulsant levels (e.g., poor compliance, increased fetal utilization, poor protein binding)
- Migraines improve in early pregnancy, exacerbate during third trimester
- Pseudotumor cerebri is more common during pregnancy
- Eclampsia of pregnancy: New-onset grand mal seizures caused by endothelial dysfunction/vascular reactivity due to immunologic reaction to placental cells
- Chorea gravidarum may occur as an exacerbation of Sydenham's chorea; represents reactivation streptococcus on the basal ganglia
- Myasthenia gravis may transiently worsen during pregnancy
- Multiple sclerosis is unchanged during pregnancy; possible increase in exacerbations during the 6 wk after parturition
- Increased incidence of carpal tunnel syndrome during pregnancy and clears after delivery; peroneal palsy may result from stirrups during delivery
- Aneurysms may enlarge during pregnancy and are more prone to rupture
- Meningiomas, AVMs may enlarge during pregnancy resulting in hemorrhage
- Sheehan's syndrome: Enlargement of preexisting pituitary tumors resulting in hemorrhagic necrosis at parturition with panhypopituitarism and blindness

Differential Dx

- Stroke
- Seizure
- Migraine
- Pseudotumor cerebri
- Eclampsia
- Posterior reversible encephalopathy syndrome
- Myasthenia gravis
- Carpal tunnel syndrome
- Multiple sclerosis
- Chorea gravidarum
- Meningioma
- AVM
- Sheehan's syndrome
- Aneurysmal rupture

Presentation/Signs & Symptoms

- Sheehan's syndrome: Severe visual impairment, headache
- Chorea gravidarum: Dancing movements of the extremities and trunk; usually occurs during the second trimester, may last until delivery
- Eclampsia: Headache, alterations in consciousness, seizures
- The transient prothrombotic state of pregnancy may result in cortical venous infarcts, causing headache, focal neurologic disturbances, and seizures
- Nearly 50% of pregnant patients experience numbness in the median nerve distribution late in the pregnancy (paresthesias in palmar surface), likely due to fluid retention in the carpal tunnel

Diagnostic Evaluation

- Investigations should be limited due to the risk of fetal injury
- X-rays and CT scans should be avoided in pregnancy unless the fetus can be adequately shielded from radiation
- MRI has not been shown to be damaging to the fetus and may be used if necessary during pregnancy
- Lumbar puncture, EEG, EMG, and nerve conduction studies may be done in pregnancy
- In epileptic patients, antiepileptic drug levels should be measured every 6 wk, and dosages should be increased accordingly
- Eclampsia is defined as grand mal seizures occurring in a pregnant patient with preeclampsia
    - Preeclampsia is defined as BP >140/90 on two separate occasions and proteinuria >300 mg/24-h urine collection

Treatment/Management

- Drugs should be carefully checked to evaluate for contraindications in pregnancy
- In migraine patients, ergotamine must be avoided, as it causes contractions of the uterus and fetal compromise
    - Mild analgesics (e.g., acetaminophen) may be used as well as short-term courses of steroids for severe headaches
    - Low-dose β-blockers may be used
- The definitive treatment of preeclampsia and eclampsia is delivery; timing depends on the severity of disease and gestational age
    - Administer IV magnesium for seizure prophylaxis during the peri- and postpartum periods
- Carpal tunnel syndrome is treated with wrist splinting

Prognosis/Complications

- Some preexisting neurologic conditions worsen during pregnancy due to hormonal factors, weight gain, or increased blood volume
- Increased risk of seizures in epileptic women
- Fetal abnormalities occur in 2% of patients on antiepileptic medications; however, if the risk of seizure is high, antiepileptics should be continued with the addition of folic acid, which may reduce the risk of fetal abnormalities
- Chorea gravidarum is much less common than in the past, and it disappears after delivery
- 12% of fetuses acquire neonatal myasthenia due to passage of acetylcholine receptor antibodies through the placenta; normally clears within 2 wk
- Eclampsia results in increased risks of stroke, hemorrhage, arteriopathy, and thrombosis
- Carpal tunnel syndrome relieved postpartum

Index

Index

Index

Index

Index

Index

Index

Index

Index

Index

Index

Index

Index

Index

Index

Index

Index